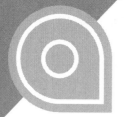

MYplace
FOR BIBLE STUDY

Published by First Place for Health
Galveston, Texas, USA
www.firstplaceforhealth.com
Printed in the USA

All Scripture quotations (unless otherwise marked) are taken from the Holy Bible, New International Version®. Copyright ©1973, 1978, 1984 by International Bible Society. Used by permission of Zondervan Publishing House.

Scripture quotations marked NLT are taken from the Holy Bible, New Living Translation. Copyright ©1996, 2004, 2007 by Tyndale House Foundation. Used by permission of Tyndale House Publishers, Inc., Carol Stream, Illinois 60188. All rights reserved.

Scripture quotations marked The Message are taken from The Message. Copyright© by Eugene H. Peterson 1993, 1994, 1995, 1996, 2000, 2001, 2002. Used by permission of NavPress Publishing Group.

Scripture quotations marked TPT are from The Passion Translation®. Copyright ©2017, 2018 by Passion & Fire Ministries, Inc. Used by permission. All rights reserved. ThePassionTranslation.com.

Scripture quotations marked AMP are taken from the Amplified® Bible. Copyright ©2015 by The Lockman Foundation, La Habra, California 90631. Used by permission. www.Lockman.org.

© 2021 First Place for Health
All rights reserved

ISBN: 978-1-942425-43-4

CONTENTS

MY PLACE FOR BIBLE STUDY
God My Refuge

Foreword by Vicki Heath 4
About the Author / About the Contributors 5
Introduction 7

Week One: A Refuge of Abundance 9
Week Two: A Refuge of Truth 26
Week Three: A Refuge of Humility 43
Week Four: A Refuge of Healing 63
Week Five: A Refuge of Mercy 84
Week Six: A Refuge of Forgiveness 100
Week Seven: A Refuge of Acceptance 121
Week Eight: A Refuge of Joy 138
Week Nine: A Time to Celebrate 155

Leader Discussion Guide 157
Jump Start Menus and Recipes 161
Steps for Spiritual Growth 183
   God's Word for Your Life 183
   Establishing a Quiet Time 185
   Sharing Your Faith 188
First Place for Health Member Survey 191
Personal Weight and Measurement Record 193
Weekly Prayer Partner Forms 195
Live It Trackers 213
100-Mile Club 231
Let's Count Our Miles 233

FOREWORD

I was introduced to First Place for Health in 1993 by my mother-in-law, who had great concern for the welfare of her grandchildren. I was overweight and overwrought! God used that first Bible study to start me on my journey to health, wellness, and a life of balance.

Our desire at First Place for Health is for you to begin that same journey. We want you to experience the freedom that comes from an intimate relationship with Jesus Christ and witness His love for you through reading your Bible and through prayer. To this end, we have designed each day's study (which will take about fifteen to twenty minutes to complete) to help you discover the deep truths of the Bible. Also included is a weekly Bible memory verse to help you hide God's Word in your heart. As you start focusing on these truths, God will begin a great work in you.

At the beginning of Jesus' ministry, when He was teaching from the book of Isaiah, He said to the people, "The Spirit of the Lord is on me, because he has anointed me to preach good news to the poor. He has sent me to proclaim freedom for the prisoners and recovery of sight for the blind, to release the oppressed, to proclaim the year of the Lord's favor" (Luke 4:18-19). Jesus came to set us free—whether that is from the chains of compulsivity, addiction, gluttony, overeating, under eating, or just plain unbelief. It is our prayer that He will bring freedom to your heart so you may experience abundant life.

God bless you as you begin this journey toward a life of liberty.

Vicki Heath, First Place for Health National Director

ABOUT THE AUTHOR

Debbie Behling joined First Place (the original name for First Place for Health) in 1981 at Houston's First Baptist Church. She became a leader the following year, and she has started groups in two other places in Texas. Currently she leads a group at Sugar Land Methodist Church in Texas, which has been meeting since 2005.

Debbie taught middle school social studies for 19 years and high school social studies online for 11 years. For 15 years she worked as an education specialist with Region 4 Education Service Center, creating numerous professional development sessions and presenting at local, state, national, and international conferences. She authored, co-authored, and/or edited over 30 publications for Region 4 between 2003 and 2018. In 2020 Debbie authored The Joy Adventure Bible study for First Place for Health.

Debbie earned a B.A. from Dallas Baptist College in 1977 with a triple major in secondary education, history, and psychology. Her postgraduate degree is a M.Ed. with a focus on educational technology from Northwestern University in Natchitoches, Louisiana.

In 2018 she retired from full-time employment in education after 35 years of teaching middle school and high school social studies and serving as an education specialist, writer, and professional development provider. She lives in Sugar Land, Texas with her husband and brood of miniature dachshunds. She has two children and one grandson. She loves to lead her First Place for Health group, write, sing in the church choir, scrapbook, travel, and research genealogy.

ABOUT THE CONTRIBUTOR

Lisa Lewis, who provided the menus and recipes in this study, is the author of *Healthy Happy Cooking*. Lisa's cooking skills have been a part of First Place for Health wellness weeks and other events for many years. She provided recipes for seventeen of the First Place for Health Bible studies and is a contributing author in *Better Together* and *Healthy Holiday Living*. She partners with community networks, including the Real Food Project, to bring healthy cooking classes to underserved areas. She is dedicated to bringing people together around the dinner table with healthy, delicious meals that are easy to prepare. Lisa lives in Galveston and is married to John. They have three children: Tal, Hunter, and Harper. Visit www.healthyhappycook.com for more delicious inspiration.

INTRODUCTION

First Place for Health is a Christ-centered health program that emphasizes balance in the physical, mental, emotional, and spiritual areas of life. The First Place for Health program is meant to be a daily process. As we learn to keep Christ first in our lives, we will find that He is the One who satisfies our hunger and our every need.

This Bible study is designed to be used in conjunction with the First Place for Health program but can be beneficial for anyone interested in obtaining a balanced lifestyle. The Bible study has been created in a seven-day format, with the last two days reserved for reflection on the material studied. Keep in mind that the ultimate goal of studying the Bible is not only for knowledge but also for application and a changed life. Don't feel anxious if you can't seem to find the correct answer. Many times, the Word will speak differently to different people, depending on where they are in their walk with God and the season of life they are experiencing. Be prepared to discuss with your fellow First Place for Health members what you learned that week through your study.

There are some additional components included with this study that will be helpful as you pursue the goal of giving Christ first place in every area of your life:

- **Leader Discussion Guide:** This discussion guide is provided to help the First Place for Health leader guide a group through this Bible study. It includes ideas for facilitating a First Place for Health class discussion for each week of the Bible study.

- **Jump Start Recipes:** There are seven days of recipes--breakfast, lunch and dinner-- to get you started.

- **Steps for Spiritual Growth:** This section will provide you with some basic tips for how to memorize Scripture and make it a part of your life, establish a quiet time with God each day, and share your faith with others..

- **First Place for Health Member Survey:** Fill this out and bring it to your first meeting. This information will help your leader know your interests and talents.

- **Personal Weight and Measurement Record:** Use this form to keep a record of your weight loss. Record any loss or gain on the chart after the weigh-in at each week's meeting.

- **Weekly Prayer Partner Forms:** Fill out this form before class and place it into a basket during the class meeting. After class, you will draw out a prayer request form, and this will be your prayer partner for the week. Try to call or email the person sometime before the next class meeting to encourage that person.

- **100-Mile Club:** A worthy goal we encourage is for you to complete 100 miles of exercise during your twelve weeks in First Place for Health. There are many activities listed on pages 265-266 that count toward your goal of 100 miles and a handy tracker to track your miles.

- **Live It Trackers:** Your Live It Tracker is to be completed at home and turned in to your leader at your weekly First Place for Health meeting. The Tracker is designed to help you practice mindfulness and stay accountable with regard to your eating and exercise habits.

WEEK ONE: A REFUGE OF ABUNDANCE

SCRIPTURE MEMORY VERSE
Since, then, you have been raised with Christ, set your hearts on things above, where Christ is, seated at the right hand of God. Colossians 3:1

Mayra had a terrible day. She forgot to set her alarm clock and was late to work. The kids left their lunches on the kitchen table. Her boss criticized her in front of her coworkers for something she didn't do. The person working with her on a time-sensitive project got called in to jury duty and would be out for at least a week. She spilled coffee on her new white shirt. And she ran out of gas on the freeway going home. All she wanted at the end of this day was a place where she could find refuge: protection from the storms of life and a soothing place of rest.

When she got home, her husband had fixed dinner and put up the laundry. Their kids were finishing their homework and eager to share their days with her. After baths and bedtime stories, she relaxed on the couch with her favorite book and cup of tea. Mayra heaved a big sigh of relief, and the stress and strain of the day melted away. She knew she would be challenged again tomorrow, but for tonight she could find refuge in the warmth of her home and family.

A refuge – a place where we can find protection from whatever is threatening us. It is often hard to find in a world filled with strife and uncertainty. We all need a place where we know we can be safe and receive comfort. For those who follow Christ, we find our refuge in God, Who provides all we need. His refuge is filled with calm, peace, and joy.

During the *God My Refuge* study, we will examine aspects of God's protection and provision. We will acquire tools to help us abide in His refuge. We will also look at false refuges, places we may go in an attempt to protect ourselves but that fall short of God's true protection. Our goal is to depend on Him alone for all that we need, because He alone provides the refuge that can save and satisfy us.

—— DAY 1: GOD'S REFUGE

My Father, how good and pleasant it is to be in Your presence. It is a holy and sacred place that fills my soul with light. Speak to me, I pray, as I open Your Word, the source of all truth.

The Bible talks about God being our *refuge* or *stronghold*, a place of protection or strength. Let's look at two examples of literal refuges or strongholds in the Old Testament. Read 1 Samuel 23:7-8 and 14. Why did Saul think he could capture David when he was in Keilah (verses 7-8)?

_____
_____
_____

The first type of refuge is one that is *man-made*. Cities in this time and place needed strong walls to protect them from invasion. Why did David escape to the desert strongholds (verse 14)?

_____
_____

The second type of refuge was part of David's *environment*, existing naturally. The Hebrew word translated "stronghold" is *misgav*. It means a high or inaccessible place, a refuge, a defense, or high fortress. It appears more than fifty times in the Bible. The most common reference is to an area where a man-made structure is erected to defend it from invaders. The purpose of the stronghold was to provide safety and protection; intruders would have a difficult time scaling or knocking down its walls.

Read 2 Samuel 5:6-7 and 9; the refuge here is translated "the fortress" in the NIV. What city did David capture, and what did he call it?

_____
_____

There was another reason for areas of protection under the Mosaic Law. Read Numbers 35:6-15. What was the purpose for the six cities of refuge?

_____
_____
_____

Finally, look at Nehemiah 12:44; the Israelites who had returned from exile finished building the walls of Jerusalem. What did they put into the storehouses within the stronghold's walls?

___

These fortresses held necessary supplies for defending the city. The fuller the storehouse, the better the stronghold could survive an attack. These purposes for a stronghold centered on protection. In light of these literal refuges, read the following verses and identify how God serves as our refuge or stronghold.

2 Samuel 22:2-3

___

Psalm 9:9

___

Psalm 27:1

___

Our God is our refuge, strength, and protection from all of life's storms. He guards us from the enemies that seek our destruction. We can rest peacefully knowing that God is for us. No matter what the world or the enemy does to us, God never leaves us. And spoiler alert: He has already won! We only need to trust Him and follow Him completely.

What is one area of your life that needs God's protection right now?

___

Close your quiet time by thanking God for His refuge. Write a prayer of gratitude for God's protection and strength, for surrounding you with His angels and keeping watch over you.

_____
_____
_____
_____
_____

Thank You, my Father, for protecting me, for being with me when I am under attack, for never leaving me, and for loving me. Amen.

—— DAY 2: SCARCITY VERSUS ABUNDANCE MINDSET
Precious Father, I come into Your blessed presence now through the gift of Jesus' sacrifice. What an honor to spend time with You today; I seek Your face to know You more.

In March 2020 a deadly virus caused shut-down and quarantine. COVID-19 caused great concern, and many restrictions were put in place to help prevent its spread. As people went to stores to stock up on supplies, a strange phenomenon took place. Toilet paper became very hard to find. For some reason, people were afraid they would run out and bought baskets full of this household staple. Grocery shelves were bare, and when a delivery of toilet paper arrived, it was snatched up quickly. Stores had to put limits on how many packages of toilet paper one person could buy. The fear of not having toilet paper during a pandemic caused people to act in bizarre ways.

When we are afraid, we will not have what we need, we may panic. We might hoard something, waiting for the perfect time to use it. We may have a large supply of what we need, more than we might use for years. This fear may be justified, but most of the time, it's likely that we overcompensate due to anxiety. Food can be one of those things we may fear will be scarce, and we may develop poor eating habits due to distress. Or we may eat to comfort ourselves when we are afraid.

Understanding the truth about God our refuge provides freedom from fear. One aspect of God's refuge is His extravagance and His desire to meet all our needs. He has a vast supply that will never run out, and He wants to give His children the very best. His shelves are never empty, and we will always be satisfied with His refuge of abundance. What does Psalm 50:10 tell us about God's supply?

_____
_____

God wants to supply all our needs. Even if we are convinced of God's sufficiency, we may feel that we are lacking. We may believe we do not have the power or capacity to meet the challenges in life, such as family relationships, job pressures, or healthy choices. This idea that we are not good enough is a mental weapon used by the enemy to keep us from freedom in Christ. This lie can also develop into a scarcity mindset where we fixate on what we don't have rather than what we do have. Turn to Exodus 16:2-3. How did the Israelites reflect a scarcity mindset?

_____
_____

In verses 4-5 and 8, how did God respond to their grumbling?

_____
_____

For years, God provided manna to the Israelites. They didn't have to farm the land to harvest it nor store up and carry food through the wilderness. It was enough to sustain them every day and it was miraculous. But the Israelites' grumbling reflects a scarcity mindset, and it continued throughout their trip between Egypt and the Promised Land. Read Numbers 11:4-6; how does this passage reflect the Israelites' scarcity mindset?

_____
_____

Did you notice that they were still obsessed with the food they ate in Egypt? They left Egypt physically, but in their minds and hearts they were still there. They took their scarcity mindset with them on the road to Canaan. The scarcity mindset says, "I can't trust God; He isn't enough." But God had begun their Exodus journey with an important principle; read Exodus 14:13-14. When they were seemingly trapped between the Egyptian army and the Red Sea, what did Moses tell them to do?

_____
_____
_____

God was enough to save them from the enemy. When my mind tells me that my circumstances are too much for me, that I am not capable of winning the battles of my life, I can reject those thoughts, standing firm in the knowledge that God my refuge is more than enough. My righteousness is not based on my own feeble attempts at holiness; Jesus is enough to cleanse me and make me whole. Instead of a scarcity mindset, I want to develop an *abundance mindset*. I know my God can part the seas and provide what I need in the wilderness. Look up Psalm 66:8-12; after many difficulties, where did the Lord bring His people?

Author Carlos Whittaker suggests a practice that may help us change from a scarcity mindset to an abundance mindset. "When Jesus prayed, He never prayed the problem....He always *prayed the promise*."[1] What would that look like for me? Perhaps instead of praying, "God, I am tired of fighting my food cravings and my weight problems; I'll never be able to change," I might pray using Romans 8:35-37: "Thank You, God, that I am more than a conqueror through Christ Who saves me, and that You will never leave me or forsake me. I trust You to help me with my eating and weight issues." Let's try it; write a sentence prayer that includes a promise from His Word.

Through his struggles with debilitating anxiety, God taught Carlos to adopt an abundance mindset. He wrote, "Abundance has nothing to do with accumulating things and everything to do with accessing the King."[2] When we access King Jesus, we have more than we need. "Jesus didn't die on a cross so we can cope!"[3] He came to give us abundant life! His victory over sin and death invites us into God's refuge of abundance.

Forgive me, dear Lord, for the times I have chosen a scarcity mindset. I know that You want to give me all I need to become all You created me to be. Thank You for Your abundant love. Amen.

—— DAY 3: GOD'S EXTRAVAGANCE
What a joy to spend time with You, my Lord. Use Your Word to lay bare my heart and reveal my innermost thoughts and motives. Cleanse and restore me through Your Spirit's power.

Yesterday we looked at developing an abundance mindset because God has all that we need. How do we go about accessing God's overflowing supply? Read Matthew 7:7-8; what three things does Jesus tell us to do?

_____
_____

In the Greek these verses have the idea of continually asking, seeking, and knocking. Some theologians think of these three actions as cumulative; first we pray (ask), then we investigate to find the truth of God's will (seek), then we are ready to take action and follow His guidance (knock). God wants us to be persistent in our requests to Him, because He has much to give us. Read verses 9-11; how do we know God's intentions toward us are to give us His best?

_____
_____
_____

When people brought problems to Jesus, His response reflected God's extravagance. Let's look at three examples. Read John 2:1-3. What problem did Mary bring to Jesus

_____
_____

How did Jesus solve the problem (verses 4-8)?

_____
_____

What was the result of Jesus' solution (verses 9-10)?

_____
_____
_____

A second story of God's extravagance is found in Luke 5. Read verses 1-5; what was the fishermen's problem?

_____
_____

What did Jesus tell the fishermen to do to solve their problem?

_____
_____

What was the result of Jesus' solution (verses 6-7)?

_____
_____

Matthew 14:13-21 reveals a third example of God's extravagance. What was the problem in verse 15?

_____
_____
_____

How did Jesus solve the problem (verses 17-19)?

_____
_____
_____

What was the result of Jesus' solution (verses 20-21)?

_____
_____
_____

In all three of these stories, the problem was brought to Jesus, and He had the solution. The solutions were not at all what the people expected! The finest wine from water, more fish than two boats could hold, and enough fish and bread to satisfy everyone with twelve baskets left over. When Jesus provides the solutions to our problems, He gives us more than we can imagine. How is that phenomenon described in Philippians 4:19?

_____
_____
_____

What does "His riches in glory in Christ Jesus" mean to you? How has God blessed you in extravagant ways?

_____
_____
_____

Read Ephesians 3:20; how does this verse reflect God's extravagance?

_____
_____
_____

What need do you have today that could use an outpouring of God's extravagance?

_____
_____
_____

As you present the problem to God and wait for His solution, remember that He is at work and will answer you with "His riches in glory in Christ Jesus." He can provide the resources you need to plan healthy meals. He provides support for making healthy choices through your team members in your First Place for Health group. Through His Spirit, He can motivate you to put Him first and follow the wellness guidelines of the First Place for Health program. He has everything we need and is willing and eager to pour out His riches on us.

Thank You, Father God, for your extravagance in my life. You lavish Your riches in glory on me, and I'm thankful I'm a child of the King. My heart rejoices in the abundance of Your supply. Amen.

—— DAY 4: THE SUFFICIENCY OF GOD'S WORD
Your Word is a lamp for my feet and a light for my path, dear God. As I open Your Word speak to my mind, appeal to my heart, and fill me with the light of Your presence.

God's Word reveals the abundance God our refuge has in store for those who seek and follow Him. What is your favorite verse or passage in the Bible? Why?

_____
_____
_____

No matter what situation we face, God's Word is more than enough to give us what we need. Read 2 Timothy 3:16-17; what can God's Word do for us?

_____
_____

As we have examined strongholds, we learned that supplies are stored in them. Weapons are also part of those supplies for protecting the strongholds. God's Word is our spiritual nourishment for our souls and our powerful tool for battle. As we read it daily and study it consistently, God's Word supplies us with an abundance of His power, power to give us what we need to make healthy choices and love Him with our whole beings. Read the scriptures below and record how God's Word supplies and empowers us.

SCRIPTURE	HOW GOD'S WORD SUPPLIES/EMPOWERS
Isaiah 55:10-11	
Matthew 24:25	
John 15:3	
John 15:7	
2 Thessalonians 2:13	

How are you currently interacting with God's Word on a regular basis?
_____
_____
_____

What is your favorite part about being involved in God's Word? Why?
_____
_____

What is your greatest challenge with engaging with God's Word? Why?
_____
_____

God's Word has been the single thing in my life than has brought the most change and satisfaction. Reading through it every year since I first joined First Place in 1981, memorizing scriptures, and studying it not just a routine for me. God's Word defines me. The power of the Word brings victory in abundance for the glory of God. One year as I began reading in Genesis in January, the Spirit focused my attention on the ways God offered mercy to his people when they rebelled against Him. He showed me how that theme repeated through the Old Testament stories. I really needed to hear that message that particular year: to receive mercy and to offer mercy to myself and others.

Thank You for Your Word, Lord, for its truth and power. Encourage me as I read, memorize, and study it. Use Your Word in my life as I face challenges and win victories in Your Name. May it live and work in me today. Amen.

—— DAY 5: ABUNDANT LIVING

As we meet together now, gracious Lord, I want to know You more. As you speak to me, may my soul, mind, heart, and body be completely open to Your Spirit's moving.

God our refuge is a place of abundance. The rich supply He provides results in abundant living, as described by Jesus in John 10:10: "I came so that they would have life, and have it abundantly." (NASB) The Greek word translated "abundantly" in this verse is *perisson*, which carries the idea of an amount so great it cannot be contained and is more than expected.

What does an abundant life look like and how do our lives overflow with the abundance of God? Read John 17:3; how is abundant life described here?

_____
_____
_____

"Eternal" is more about quality than quantity. A life centered on knowing God is a rich life, no matter how long it lasts. It is not about an abundance of possessions, status, or power. It is about an abundance of God living in and through us. It is the richness of God in us, not the wealth of the world for us. Read Colossians 3:1, this week's memory verse. Write it here and practice your memorization.

_____
_____
_____

This verse tells us an important part of developing a mindset of abundance. It is about where we focus our thoughts: "things above." Interestingly, the Greek word translated "above" not only means located in a higher place but can also carry the idea of "to the brim," another connection to abundance. And we focus on "things above" because we "have been raised with Christ." He is above us, "seated at the right hand of God." Therefore, our focus should be on Him, the One with Whom we have been raised.

Paul was one who lived an abundant life. He talked about his experiences in 2 Corinthians 11:23-28. He was defending his apostleship because of some accusations. Read these verses and summarize Paul's life as he described it.

_____
_____
_____

Paul explained his life's goal in Philippians 3:10-12. Identify what Paul wanted to gain.

_____
_____

In 2 Timothy 4:6-8 Paul looked back on his life and gave a final assessment and his future hope. What did he say?

_____
_____
_____

Paul's life reveals these things about abundant living.
- Knowing God is the greatest source of abundant life.
- An abundant mindset is concerned about things of eternal rather than temporal value.
- There are both positive and negative experiences in an abundant life.
- Abundant living is a process that lasts a lifetime and reaps eternal rewards.

Abundance is not in what we have but Who has us. A God-centered life is an abundant life because the things of this world are put in their proper perspective, and the future hope of living forever with Him motivates everything we desire and do. An abundant life is not an easier life, but it is a satisfying life, filled to the brim and overflowing.

Thank You, God, for the abundance of living You provide through Your Son Jesus. Help me to embrace both the power of the resurrection and the fellowship of suffering that I have in Him. Focus my thoughts on things above where He is seated at Your right hand. You are my all in all. Amen.

—— DAY 6: REFLECTION AND APPLICATION

In these quiet moments with You, my Lord, I seek Your heart. I am still and listening for Your sweet whispers and Spirit movement in me, knowing Your love for Me is endless.

In 2 Kings 13:10-19, we find a story about the prophet Elisha. Verses 10-13 give us the context: Israel's King Jehoash was dead after 16 years of an evil rule. His son Jeroboam was the new king. In verse 14 he went to visit Elisha. What was the situation?

What did Elisha tell King Jeroboam to do in verses 15-17? Why?

Elisha told King Jeroboam to do something else in verse 18; what was it and how did the king respond?

What did Elisha say in verse 19?

King Jeroboam lost an opportunity to totally defeat his enemy. What does this story teach us about God's abundance and our access to it?

- Even though the king was not a true follower of God, He wanted to give total victory to him. He was another in a long line of Israelite rulers who worshiped idols instead of being completely devoted to Yahweh. Yet God kept His covenant with His people despite their rebellion. Even though we don't always follow God completely, He still offers victory to us.
- God offered King Jeroboam the opportunity to completely defeat his enemy. But He wanted to test his faith in God's promise of victory. After Elisha showed him a direct connection between the arrows and God's deliverance, the king only struck the ground with the arrows three times. He re-vealed his lack of faith in God's abundance. If he had struck the ground many times, God would have given him total victory rather than partial victory. God invites us to engage with Him in receiving the abundance He has planned for us. How enthusiastic are we? How strongly do we believe in His provisions? He wants to see us respond to Him boldly, anticipating all the ways He will provide for and bless us.

God is limitless; we need to be careful not to limit Him by lack of faith. We may put parameters around God, only allowing Him to work in our lives in some areas and not others. What a blessing we miss when we do that. He eagerly waits to pour out more than we can ask or think if we will believe and live in the light of that truth. 2 Peter 1:3-4 says, "His divine power has given us *everything we need* for a godly life through our knowledge of him who called us by his own glory and goodness. Through these he has given us his very great and precious promises, so that through them you may participate in the divine nature, having escaped the corruption in the world caused by evil desires."

Write a prayer acknowledging God's abundance and asking Him to show you where you may be limiting Him. Ask Him for help to believe and be enthusiastic about what He wants to pour out on you. Thank Him for His sufficiency and love.

Thank You for Your amazing abundance, Lord, and Your desire to give me an unending supply of Your deliverance. Help my faith in You to grow and give me enthusiasm for the future as I contemplate Your love for me. I am Yours, Father, and I love You. Amen.

—— DAY 7: REFLECTION AND APPLICATION

Thank You for this week's study, dear Father. I want to live out the truths You are teaching me. As I reflect on those truths, give me deeper insight into Who You are and who I am in light of them.

Each week we end our study with a time of personal reflection. It is just that: your own personal thoughts, questions, and meditations on God and what He is specifically saying to you. You choose how you will process your reflection; here are some guidelines.

- There is no one way or a "right" way to spend this time reflecting. You decide what meets your needs.
- You can listen to Christian music, write in a journal, or sit quietly and listen to God speak to you.
- You may go back and re-read one or more of the scripture passages from this week's study and meditate on them.
- You may take a walk and concentrate on the beauty of nature as you reflect.
- Whatever your chosen mode of reflection, use this time to review what God is teaching you and ask Him to apply it to you personally.

You may want to jot down some notes about your reflections each week. There is space below for you to do that. If you would like to go further with journaling, there are some optional prompts below to help you get started. This activity is not homework or required; do whatever God leads you to do to meet your needs.

If you choose to journal, it could take various forms and should be whatever suits you best. You may choose to create a journal just for this study. Use paper or a digital method. Write in this Bible study book or another journal. Use words, images, or both. Record your voice on your digital device. Use one format or multiple formats; any format is good if it works for you.

Optional Journaling Prompts (choose one)
- Keep a record of the scripture verses that relate to finding God as your refuge. Write reflections on any that you wish.
- Record quotes from the Bible, this Bible study, and/or other sources that encourage you, challenge you, or inspire you in this process of experiencing God as your refuge. Here's one to get you start-ed: "Any refuge other than God is probably something that I should seek refuge from rather than seek refuge in." (Craig D. Lounsbrough)

MYplace O FOR BIBLE STUDY

- Locate images that relate to your faith walk and put them in your journal. You can pair them with quotes or your own words. The images could form a collage to which you add throughout this study and beyond. For this week's study, you might locate an image of a stronghold that would have existed during the time that David was king.
- Take any idea or activity from this week's lesson and go deeper. Look for more resources that re-late to that concept, and record how it relates to you. For example, you could write more prayers with promises rather than problems as we did on Day 2.
- Find a song that encourages you in this process. You may document the lyrics and record your own reflections on them, or you could illustrate them with sketches or images you locate. Two examples for this week's study are "God of Abundance" by Ayo Davies (2018) or "Abundantly More" by Seth Condrey (2018).

Your journal is a very private and personal process; therefore, share it carefully. If social media is a healthy place for you, use these hashtags for posting your words, images, or other reflections or personal stories from this study: #fp4h and #fp4hgodmyrefuge. You can view my journal and others' entries using these hashtags.

May I pray over you as together we consider God our refuge? Please put your name in the blanks below. Consider saying the prayer aloud and repeat it whenever you desire.

Most loving and holy Father, thank You for _____ and that _____ joined this First Place for Health study at this time in this place for Your purposes. Bless _____ as _____ faces the coming weeks. _____ has needs that only Your refuge of love can satisfy. Protect _____'s schedule so _____ will regularly have time alone with You and Your Word. Guard _____ from the enemy, who has no authority over _____, because Your Spirit lives in _____ and Your Son Jesus has won _____'s victory over all. We thank You and praise You now for the amazing way You are working in _____. May _____ walk in your mercy and grace as, with Your help, _____ lives in You, the only perfect and complete refuge, in Your Name and for Your glory. Amen.

Your Journaling:

Notes

1. Carlos Whittaker, Enter Wild: Exchange a Mild and Mundane Faith for Life with an Uncontainable God (Colorado Springs, CO: Waterbrook, 2020), 74.
2. Ibid, 19.
3. Ibid, 71.

WEEK TWO: A REFUGE OF TRUTH

SCRIPTURE MEMORY VERSE
The Lord is a refuge for the oppressed, a stronghold in times of trouble.
Psalm 9:9

Helen Baratta, First Place for Health Director of Development, has an amazing story. After joining First Place for Health, she lost over 100 pounds and has maintained her weight loss for many years. In her success story, she recounts her struggle with obesity.

> At the age of 35, no longer able to hide from myself that I was obese, I gave up and moved onto other priorities in life. Aside from this struggle, I had a lot to be thankful for, including a wonderful husband, Vince, who loves me just as I am, fat or thin. His career as a contract engineer had us relocating all over the country, and with each impending move, I lost weight then gained it back after we settled in a new location. It was fun to reinvent our lives with each relocation, but this issue of being overweight followed me wherever we went. In spite of being loved and supported by Vince and other friends and family members, I felt powerless. Like so many others who struggle with weight, I tried everything: starvation in college, Weight Watchers before my wedding, diet pills after my first child, and Weight Watchers again after my second child when the scale tipped over 200 pounds.[1]

Perhaps you can relate to Helen's predicament. Like Helen, you may find that "My weight chart looked like the Dow Jones: up, down, up, up, down, up, up, down and always back up no matter what I tried." This roller coaster ride is often indicative of a deeper conflict in one's life: a past trauma, a learned behavioral pattern, or some intense, unfulfilled need. The conflict and pain has caused the creation of a protective wall which defends against hurt but prevents healing.

These self-protecting walls can keep us from resolving conflicts; they can also separate us from God. They create a false refuge, a place we go for comfort that only keeps us from the Healer we need. When we go to God for refuge instead of food or other temporary comforts, we find what we really need. Only He can truly satisfy us and give us freedom and peace.

Last week in "A Refuge of Abundance," we explored these truths.
- God is our refuge or stronghold, providing safety and supply.
- We can develop an abundance mindset rather than a scarcity mindset, trusting God will provide everything we need.
- God has an extravagant supply that we can access by persistently asking, knocking, and seeking Him.
- God's Word is sufficient for sustaining us and empowering us through His Spirit.
- The abundant life is achieved by knowing God, full of ups and downs, focused on the eternal rather than the temporal, and a life-long process that reaps eternal rewards.

This week we will examine God's authentic refuge compared to false refuges. As you seek God this week, ask Him to show you how He is your refuge and pray for His help in giving you victory over any false refuge you may have. It is a first step in stopping the seemingly never-ending weight gain/loss/gain cycle.

—— DAY 1: GOD'S TRUE REFUGE

My Father, how good and pleasant it is to be in Your presence. It is a holy and sacred place that fills my soul with light. Speak to me, I pray, as I open Your Word, the source of all truth.

Our memory verse for this week is from Psalm 9:9. Write it here.
_____
_____
_____

Notice that both "refuge" and "stronghold" are used in this verse. They are similar in meaning in the Bible, as we saw last week. Abiding in God's true refuge has some amazing benefits. Read Psalm 62:5-8 in the NIV version and analyze David's poem about God as his refuge.

Verse 5: David's soul waits in _____ for God alone, for his _____ is from Him.

Verse 6: God alone is David's _____ and his _____, his _____; he will not be _____.

MYplace O FOR BIBLE STUDY

Verse 7: David's _____ and his _____ rest on God; the _____ of his _____, his _____ is in God.

Verse 8: _____ in Him at all times, you people; _____ out your _____ before Him; God is a _____ for us.

What images does David use to describe God in these verses?
_____
_____
_____

David looks to God to find something; what is it
_____
_____
_____

What does Proverbs 18:10 tell us about the refuge of God?
_____
_____
_____

Read Psalm 46:1-3; because God is my refuge, what can I do?
_____
_____
_____

How has God been your refuge? Give one example of how He has protected and provided for you.
_____
_____
_____

God's true refuge is our only real source of strength, protection, and deliverance. When we know God more, we recognize the false refuge that may seek to replace Him. We'll begin to look at those tomorrow. For today, let's thank God for His protection, and like David in Psalm 62:5, let us wait in silence for God alone, for our hope is from Him. Write a prayer expressing your thoughts and feelings to God about Him being your true refuge.

I praise You, dear God, for Your unshakeable strength and thank You that I can depend on You for protection and provision. No matter what challenges are before me, I can rest within Your refuge, hoping in You alone. Amen.

—— DAY 2: A FALSE REFUGE INSTEAD OF GOD'S REFUGE

Hello, dear Father. I come before You now and thank You for Your love and care for me. Open my eyes as I study Your Word so I can drink in all its richness.

God is our refuge, a place of protection. But sometimes we choose a personal refuge or stronghold, replacing God's perfect plan with our own designs. The enemy is in the business of taking what God creates for good and manipulating it for his own purposes. He wants us to build a personal refuge, a counterfeit to replace God's perfect protection. We may subconsciously erect a stronghold for temporary protection, but it may eventually imprison us, not protect us. This false refuge may cause a pattern or habit that characterizes our behavior. That is not what Jesus wants for us. Read John 10:10 and fill in the blanks below.

    Jesus wants us to have _____.
    The enemy wants to _____.

What does the last part of Isaiah 28:15 say?

_____
_____
_____

Food is one example of this phenomenon. In itself, food is vital to our existence. God created all food to be good for us to eat (Genesis 1-2), fuel our bodies, and bring pleasure. But we can take God's good creation and create a false refuge. Let's begin by asking some questions as we consider the role that food plays in our lives. When you make unhealthy choices, what do you believe is your motivation? What do you think triggers uncontrollable urges?

_____
_____
_____

We may be using food to avoid change, to keep us from confronting pain and finding healing. This pattern of behavior started for me on the day I turned six years old. My parents separated on my birthday, and my mother, two younger sisters, and I went to live with her family in another state. An inner voice began to tell me that I had to be strong for my mom and sisters since my dad wasn't around. Although my parents reconciled after a few weeks, and we moved back to our home soon after, the message was planted deep within me. A six-year-old is not strong enough to care for her family; I faced an insurmountable challenge. As a result, I began to eat as a defense mechanism, as a way to comfort myself and avoid the fear and pain I was feeling. Although I was doing the best that I could do, subconsciously food began to take a "strong hold" on me. After years of this behavior, I became trapped in a prison of overeating and overweight.

As we study God our refuge, we will also look at various false refuges and how we can work alongside God to leave them behind. This study seeks to meet you where you are in at least one of these three ways.

- Your story may be similar to mine; you have some event in life that caused you to use food or another coping mechanism as a way to deal with fear and pain. Some scientific studies estimate up to 80% of the population has experienced life-altering trauma. Obsessive behaviors we use to cope with hurt can take various forms. If that is true for you, get ready for good news. Our great God is able to bring you healing and restoration! It is a process that requires work, but He is strong and mighty to save. The work you do will be worth the freedom you gain.
- You are blessed to have never experienced life-altering trauma. However, other people in your life may struggle with a false refuge born out of pain. Understanding how strongholds are created and how God can be the true refuge provides insights that He can use in your relationships with others. You can't remove the strongholds for them, but God can use you as a resource and support. You can empathize with them as they seek healing and restoration as you abide in God as your refuge.
- Keep in mind that just because you do not struggle with a false refuge now doesn't mean it can't happen in the future. Strongholds are built slowly over time. It is much easier to stop the building process than to tear down existing strongholds. Or you may have broken down a false refuge in the past and want to ensure it is not rebuilt. Be aware and work with God your refuge to prevent strongholds from forming.

One step is to ask God to reveal a false refuge we may have. What did Jesus say about the enemy in John 8:44?

What does Jesus say about the truth in John 8:32?

It is blessed to live outside a false refuge and completely within the refuge of God. Take time now to tell God your thoughts and ask Him for wisdom and courage to seek the truth about anything keeping you from totally abiding in His refuge alone.

Mighty Savior, how I need You as I seek to understand what motivates my behaviors. Thank You that You are my true refuge, for Your power to eliminate a false refuge. I trust You to work in me to bring healing and restoration, using Your truth set me free. Amen.

—— DAY 3: SOURCES OF A FALSE REFUGE: UNCONFESSED SIN AND UNFORGIVENESS

What a privilege to come into Your presence, dear Lord, where I can find rest and peace. Examine my heart and reveal my innermost secrets so I can become whole.

Yesterday we began recognizing the reality of a false refuge. Next we want to look at some of the more specific causes of a false refuge. The first two are opposite sides of the same coin: unconfessed sin and unforgiveness.[1]

Unconfessed Sin You may already practice confessing your sins to God on a regular basis. As long as we live on earth, we have the potential to struggle with sin, and we will continue to need to confess our sins to God and receive His forgiveness. Read Psalm 66:18-20 and describe the psalmist's concern about his sin.

The word "cherished" in this verse is also translated "harbored," "regarded," and "seen." There is a sense that I am looking intently at my sin. Will I keep it to myself because I cherish it, or will I bring it before God, release it, and receive His cleansing?

One of the ways the enemy manipulates our propensity to sin is to accuse us and make us doubt God's forgiveness. After you make unhealthy food choices, you may feel guilty. You may give up trying and think, "I'll never be able to eat like a normal person!" That belief can create a downward spiral of overeating and shaming. Turn to Romans 8:1-2 and write it here. Circle the words "no condemnation" and "set you free."

_____
_____
_____

Read 1 John 1:9, write it here, and circle the words "purify" and "all unrighteousness."

_____
_____
_____

Your body is God's temple, and the Holy Spirit resides there (1 Corinthians 6:19-20). Taking care of our bodies is good stewardship, and if we consistently treat ourselves in unhealthy ways, we are not good managers of God's temples. If you are bound up in a cycle of overeating, losing and gaining weight, despair, and shame, you may feel it will never end. Sweet friend, God offers you freedom through His Son Jesus that can break this cycle..

What does Romans 5:8 say about God's love for you?

_____
_____
_____

Take a moment right now to thank Him for His forgiveness and confess any sins that come to mind. Write a sentence prayer here.

_____
_____
_____

Unforgiveness God offers forgiveness to us despite our inability to live without sin. How can we accept God's grace and mercy freely but withhold that same forgiveness from those who have offended us? Read Matthew 6:12; what does that look like for you?

_____
_____
_____

Most of us know people who have refused to forgive those who have hurt them. Their lives usually become marked by bitterness and pain. Forgiveness is hard. In fact, it is impossible without God working within a person to free her from pain and the desire for revenge. It can damage other relationships, and it can be a source of inner turmoil. Turn to Romans 12:17-21; how are we to handle those who hurt us?

_____
_____
_____

Is there someone you need to forgive? Take a moment to ask God for help in releasing your hurt and anger and begin forgiving that person. Understand that forgiveness is a process, and you may need to ask God for help many times before you are delivered from a spirit of unforgiveness. Write a sentence prayer here.

_____
_____
_____

Tomorrow we will look at additional reasons we may build a false refuge that imprisons rather than protects us. These first two causes, unconfessed sin and unforgiveness, require consistent, intentional attention, processing them with God's help. Spend the rest of your quiet time with God today praying over these two areas, listening to Him as He speaks to you. Only He has the cleansing power to wipe away our sins and free us to forgive those who offend us. His refuge is free from sin and bitterness. Record any thoughts you have about your process of receiving and giving forgiveness.

_____
_____
_____

Father, I am in awe of Your forgiveness toward me. I fail to keep all Your commands, yet You are eager to pour out mercy on me. Give me the same attitude toward those who hurt me; I want to be free from holding grudges and desiring revenge. Thank You for never giving up on me. Amen.

—— DAY 4: SOURCES OF A FALSE REFUGE: LIES AND HEREDITY

As I come now into Your presence, Lord, I am in awe of Your generous grace and mercy. I have not been completely faithful to You, yet You are always faithful to me. Help me learn to trust You more as I listen to You now.

Yesterday we looked at the two-sided coin of unconfessed sin and unforgiveness, two of the reasons we might retreat to a false refuge. Today we will investigate two more sources: lies and heredity.

Lies

Imagine being jilted on your wedding day. One broken-hearted woman reacted to this tragedy in an extreme way: she wore her wedding dress every day for the rest of her life, stopped the clocks in her house at the time she was left at the altar, and kept the wedding dinner and cake out on a table, uneaten and rotting. She refused to allow any sunlight in her house, living in darkness and shadow. She wanted her life to freeze at the moment before she was betrayed. This woman is a sad character in Charles Dickens' novel Great Expectations. Her name? Miss Havisham. She was "having a sham" or living in a fake world of her own making.

We have already looked at John 8:44 where Jesus tells us that our enemy is the father of lies. Adam and Eve were the first to succumb to his deceit (Genesis 3). We are constantly confronted with opportunities to believe lies in the hopes of avoiding painful truths. Over time, these lies can create a false refuge that prevents us from honestly looking at our thoughts and behaviors, creating a barrier to God's refuge of mercy and grace.

King Saul is an unfortunate example of this condition. Read 1 Samuel 18:6-9; what did Saul believe about David?

_____
_____
_____

Now read 1 Samuel 24:1-13; what did David do that showed King Saul's beliefs about him were not true?

_____
_____
_____

David had a second opportunity to kill King Saul and again he spared him (1 Samuel 26). Saul didn't accept the truth that David was faithful to him and had no desire to take the kingdom from him. His fear and jealousy got the best of him, and he believed the lie. It became a stronghold for him that clouded his judgment and ruined his life.

What happens when we believe lies in this way? We may think we will never be successful in making healthy choices consistently. We can buy into fad diets that promise quick weight loss but don't address the reason we gained the weight in the first place. We might blame our problems on others without looking at our own actions and attitudes that contribute to our situation. Believing in these lies keep us from taking action and seeking God for help in meaningful change.

Charles Dickens' Miss Havisham went on to teach her adopted daughter to manipulate men and hurt them as she had been hurt. Living in a lie not only hurts you but others you care about. Take a minute to reflect on any lies you struggle with. Ask God to reveal them to you and record your reflection.

_____
_____
_____

Heredity

You may have behavioral patterns that you have adopted from your family of origin. Your family may have musical talents, athletic abilities, or scientific minds that show up in various people. But harmful behaviors can be passed on as well. For example, children whose parents abuse substances of any kind can seem pre-programmed to follow in their footsteps.

Let's look at an example in the Bible. Read Genesis 12:10-13. What did Abram say about his wife while they were in Egypt?

_____
_____
_____

What was the result (verses 14-20)?

___

This story is repeated in Genesis 20; Abram, now called Abraham, gave into his fear instead of trusting God and lied once again. He put his wife in danger in order to save his own skin. Not a stellar moment in his life. But the lying doesn't end with Abraham. Read Genesis 26, verses 1 and 7. What did Abraham's son Isaac do?

___

Even though Isaac was not born yet when his father Abraham twice lied about Sarah being his wife, he repeats his father's lie. And his son Jacob, with help from his mother Rebekah, carries on the family tradition of lying in Genesis 27. What does Jacob do to his own father in verses 14-19?

___

Patterns of behavior in a family can be powerful strongholds. Small children tend to mimic the people in their families of origin as they develop. Some characteristics can even be passed on to future generations through DNA. The National Institutes of Health report that "as much as half of a person's risk of becoming addicted to nicotine, alcohol, or other drugs depends on his or her genetic makeup."[2] Our inclination to sin runs deep within us. It doesn't mean that our DNA forces us to repeat familial self-destructive patterns. It does mean we have to guard against giving in to those tendencies. God provides help in overcoming our sinful predispositions. Christ died to provide forgiveness for sin, and the Holy Spirit lives in believers' hearts to guard, guide, and direct us to overcome it.

The remedy for changing each of these behaviors is to identify the root source and address it. This study provides opportunities to examine these and other false refuges and ways to abide only in God's refuge instead. For today, let us pray for God's help and thank Him for what He will do to transform us as we encounter Him in fresh ways. Write your prayer here.

_____
_____
_____
_____
_____
_____
_____
_____
_____

Father, I am learning about how a false refuge can keep me from living the abundant life Jesus came to give me. You are greater than any challenge I will encounter, and You have plans to prosper me, to give me hope and a future. I trust You to bring me closer to You. Amen.

—— DAY 5: REFUGE IN CHRIST AS MY IDENTITY
Create in me a clean heart, oh God, and renew a right spirit within me. Restore the joy of Your salvation to me, and give me a willing spirit.

A false refuge we create usually starts in our minds. We may believe a lie that affects our behavior that leads us into a false refuge. If we develop entrenched ways of thinking and feeling, it becomes a habit. The false refuge we seek to protect us from danger become dangerous itself, keeping us from God's true refuge of health and freedom.

As we explore many aspects of a false refuge, we need to be grounded in our identity in Christ. Starting with the truth will equip us to expose the lies that may be buried in our beliefs and behaviors. Read each scripture below and record what it tells you about your identity in Christ.

SCRIPTURE	MY IDENTITY IN CHRIST
Genesis 1:27	
2 Corinthians 5:17	

1 Peter 2:9	
Galatians 2:20	
John 1:12	
Ephesians 2:8-10	
John 15:15	

Spend the rest of your quiet time today deeply meditating on these passages and your identity in Christ. Here are some practical things you can do. Choose one or more of these activities.

- Read each passage aloud.
- Read one passage several times.
- Replace the pronouns with your name (e.g., "Debbie is crucified with Christ...").
- Emphasize different words each time you read the verse.
- What questions does the verse bring to your mind?
- How does this verse differ from what you currently think about yourself?
- Which characteristics are easy for you to accept? Which ones are harder?
- Record your thoughts here or in your journal.

These words of God can be an anchor for you. Consider bookmarking this page, coming back to remind yourself Whose you are and the truth He says about you. The enemy doesn't want you to focus on these truths; he wants you to believe the lies that you tell yourself and what the world says about you. Praise God we are redeemed and belong to God!

Proclaim this powerful reality from 1 John 4:4: "You, dear children, are from God and have overcome [every spirit that doesn't come from God], because the *One Who is in you is greater than the one who is in the world.*" Jesus has defeated the enemy and lives in you to free you from a false refuge. Continually claim that truth as you seek God your authentic refuge.

Thank You, Jesus, that my identity is in You and not in the world. I am Your child, Your friend, Your workmanship, Your creation, and an overcomer. May the words of my mouth and the meditation of my heart be acceptable in Your sight, for You are my Rock and my Redeemer. Amen.

—— DAY 6: REFLECTION AND APPLICATION

Father God, Your strength and power are unlimited, and I want to draw on Your supply, not depend on myself. Speak to my heart and fill me with Your Spirit as I stop and spend these moments with You.

This week we've explored truths about God our refuge and false refuges. Let's consider some steps we can take to expose a false refuge we may have and begin to address the causes.

- First, recognize the false refuge. Name it and call it what it is.
- Second, declare that it will come down, even as the demolition process is just beginning. Speak the words, "Break down this false refuge!" aloud and repeatedly; pray and thank God for what He is doing.
- Third, remember that leaving the false refuge takes time. Hard work may last for a while before results are evident; trust that God is working when progress is not apparent.
- Fourth, when the false refuge comes down, rejoice! However, remain vigilant to ensure it doesn't begin to reappear.
- Fifth, more than one false refuge may need to be destroyed. If any are left, the struggle with unhealthy behaviors may continue. Don't stop until every false refuge is vacated and you are totally abiding in God your refuge.
- Finally, trust God as you leave the false refuge behind. Hope in Him, not personal strength or abilities. Participation in the process is necessary, but God is the Source of the power and direction.

Leaving behind a false refuge is not an individual task. It requires support from others, and if you discover you don't currently have a false refuge, you can be a valuable support for someone who does. Be willing to ask your First Place for Health group members as well as other trusted family and friends to assist you in your process; if you need additional help from professionals, consider engaging a Christian counselor. The First Place for Health series, My Place for Discovery, is a powerful resource for working through the causes for unhealthy lifestyles. Pastor and author Max Lucado gives us this wise advice.

Have you asked others to help you? Everything inside you says: keep the struggle a secret. Wear a mask, hide the pain. God says just the opposite: "Make this your common practice: Confess your sins to each other and pray for each other so that you can live together whole and healed" (James 5:16 MSG). Satan indwells the domain of shadows and secrets. God lives in the land of light and honesty. Bring your problem into the open. Ask for help. Get drastic. Try a fresh approach. Who knows, you may be a prayer away from a breakthrough.[3]

Say these words aloud: "God, break down the false refuge of (name of stronghold) in my life!" For example, "God, break down the false refuge of pride in my life!" Write those words here.

God, break down the false refuge of _____ in my life!"

Say this statement aloud several times and over several days. You can change the wording to an active affirmation: "God, You are breaking down the false refuge of _____ in my life!"

Write a prayer of thanksgiving to God for what He has shown you thus far and for the eventual freedom from the false refuge. Remember "you may be a prayer away from a breakthrough."

_____
_____
_____
_____

I recognize there may be a false refuge in my life, Lord, and only You can break it down. I want to live in freedom with nothing to imprison me and keep me from healthy relationships with You, others, and myself. I thank You in advance for the deliverance and refuge You provide. Amen.

—— DAY 7: REFLECTION AND APPLICATION
God Almighty, Maker of heaven and earth, it is such joy to come into Your presence. My heart is open to the moving of Your Spirit; do Your sacred work in my mind and heart.

We started this week looking at Helen Baratta's story about her battle with weight. Listen to her remarkable words describing her victory.

I know now that *being overweight is a physical problem with a spiritual solution.* First, I learned to trust God. God accepted and loved me exactly as I was, yet cared for me and did not allow me to remain hopeless. In 2006, God brought First Place for Health into my life. As I learned a new way to place Christ first, my love for the Lord expanded. I learned to listen for and obey His promptings to get to the root of what was causing my weight issue. Every time that God helped me remove a scarred layer from my past, I embraced a new layer of trust in His plan for my life. I crawled, then walked and finally ran free from a life of obesity to one of health and hope, which has given me the strength to accomplish the goals and dreams He had planned for my life. I reached my goal in 2010 and each passing year since then has resulted in learning something new about myself. I'm not going to mislead anyone by saying that my life became perfect and easy and wonderful. Just like everyone else, I've had my share of challenges, but food is no longer my solution to coping with them.[4] (emphasis added)

Helen is an inspiring example of God's power to free us with His refuge of truth. He desires for you to live in His truth and not the lies of a false refuge. Spend your quiet time today reviewing what He is teaching you and asking for His help in revealing any lies you are believing. Here are some possible prompts to consider as you reflect.

Optional Journaling Prompts (choose one)
- Record the ways you have made progress addressing a false refuge during the week's study. How has God's Word provided insight into your false refuge? What questions do you have about your process?
- Create a two-column chart. On the left column, list lies you believe that you are uncovering or lies that the world tries to get you to believe. On the right column, list the truths you've learned about God's refuge. Thank God for His true refuge and ask for His help in trusting His truth.
- Find a photo of you with your family. Pray over yourself and the members of your family, especially any family issues past or present. Thank God for His healing power in your family's behaviors and relationships with each other.
- Find a song that encourages you in this process. You may document the lyrics and record your own reflections on them, or you could illustrate them with sketches or images you locate. Two examples are "Come And Tear Down The Walls / I Surrender All" by David Nicole Binion (2020) and the classic hymn "A Mighty Fortress is Our God" by Martin Luther.

Your journal is a very private and personal process; therefore, share it carefully. If social media is a healthy place for you, use these hashtags for posting your words, images, or other reflections or personal stories from this study: #fp4h and #fp4h-godmyrefuge. You can view my journal and others' entries using these hashtags.

My Father, You are my true refuge. No other refuge gives me peace, rest, and protection. I want to let go of any lies that keep me from experiencing You and pray for Your continued work in me to reveal lies and replace them with Your truth. Amen.

Your Journaling

Notes
[1] Helen Baratta, First Place for Health: https://www.firstplaceforhealth.com/helen-baratta/.
[2] NIDA, "Genetics and Epigenetics of Addiction Drug Facts," June 16, 2020. https://www.drugabuse.gov/publications/drugfacts/genetics-epigenetics-addiction.
[3] Max Lucado, "Strongholds," 2015. https://maxlucado.com/strongholds/.
[4] Helen Baratta, op. cit.

WEEK THREE: A REFUGE OF HUMILITY

SCRIPTURE MEMORY VERSE
Therefore, as it is written: "Let the one who boasts boast in the Lord." 1 Corinthians 1:31

Edinburgh, Scotland is home to an imposing castle. Built in the Iron Age, it has withstood thousands of years of war. Although it seems impregnable, it was once captured due to the overconfidence of its inhabitants. There is one spot that seemed too strong for anyone to capture, so it was left unguarded. The attacking army was able to capture the fort with just a small group of soldiers getting through the vulnerable area. By focusing on the weak parts of the fortress, the leaders let the strongest part become weak. As we seek to vacate a false refuge, we must not become complacent about our strengths, because they can prove to be the biggest barriers to abiding in God's refuge alone.

Last week we explored these truths about God our refuge of truth.
- God is our true refuge, a place of refuge and protection.
- We may replace God's true refuge with our own false refuge that imprisons us rather than protects us.
- A false refuge can be caused by unconfessed sin and unforgiveness of others.
- Lies that we believe and hereditary influences can lead to a false refuge.
- Learning the truth about my identity in Christ can help me recognize lies that trap me in a false refuge.

This week we will tackle what is likely our greatest enemy: pride. Pride can keep us from facing our unhealthy choices and make us defensive, not open to change. Like Edinburgh Castle, pride seem insurmountable, but we have God on our side. With Him, we are sure to conquer our pride and win our freedom to humbly live solely in God's refuge.

—— DAY 1: PRIDE AS A FALSE REFUGE

My Father, what a privilege to come before You now, to sit at Your feet, to hear Your tender voice, and to experience Your constant love. My heart is open to learn from You and enjoy Your presence.

When your child does something well, it brings a sense of pride. If you meet your goals at work, you are proud of your accomplishments. When you create something that brings joy, you feel satisfaction and pride in what you have made. These feelings of pride are normal and good. Yet pride can get out of control and keep us from depending on God as our refuge. This kind of pride can create a false refuge. Basically, any false refuge has pride at its source. It stems from an attitude that says, "I'm smart enough to figure out my life. I know what is best for me, and I don't need any help." We misplace our faith, relying on self instead of God. It is the basis for all of our sin.

Pride appears in a story in Exodus 32. The people of Israel escaped from Egypt and arrived at Mount Sinai. Moses went up the mountain to talk with God and received directions about a covenant God wanted to make with the people. What does verse 1 tell us that they decided to do while Moses was away?

_____
_____
_____

What did God have to say about the people? (verse 9)

_____
_____
_____

The Hebrew word translated "stiff-necked" in English often referred to an ox that was hitched to a plow or cart. The driver holding the reins attempted to direct the ox but it refused to comply. It held its neck stiff to prevent it from being led in a different direction. The ox chose its own path and would not yield to the driver's expertise.

What evidence did God have that the Israelites were stiff-necked? Read the following passages and identify how they resisted God's leadership and lacked faith in Him.

Verses in Exodus	The Israelites' Resistance to Gods Leadership/Lack of Faith
14:10-12	
15:22-27	
16:1-3	

WEEK THREE A REFUGE OF HUMILITY

Their stiff-necked behavior continued throughout their history. How would you summarize the Israelites' hearts and actions as God delivered them from Egyptian slavery and set them on the journey to the Promised Land?

_____
_____
_____

What warning did God give His people in Psalm 32:8-10?

_____
_____
_____

This stiff-necked syndrome is referenced in the New Testament as well. In Acts 7, Stephen recounted much of Jewish history to those who opposed Jesus' gospel. What did he say to them in verse 51?

_____
_____
_____

Circle the phrase, "resist the Holy Spirit." Here is a key to understanding the false refuge of pride. God tells us what to do through His Holy Spirit, Who lives in those who follow Christ. One of His roles in our lives is to guide us into God's truth (John 16:13). When we resist His leadership or refuse to accept His truth, we are being *stiff-necked*. Have you experienced this situation? You sense the leading of the Holy Spirit, and yet you don't want to follow. You can feel your body tightening as you try to avoid even sensing His voice. You may even feel your neck become stiff! And why would we choose to ignore the guidance of our Lord, Who loves us and has our best in mind at all times? Pride. We want to hold the reins and drive the cart. We want to do it our way.

Consider doing something practical to address this condition. Close your eyes and relax your body as much as you can. Slowly rotate your head from left to right, up and down, and in a circle, first one direction then the other. Focus on your neck, noticing any stiffness, and ask God to help you release that stiffness to Him. As you continue moving your head slowly and gently, confess any known sin to Him and receive His forgiveness. Feel the tension leave your body. End this relaxation session with your head bowed, saying a prayer of thanksgiving to God and asking Him to keep your neck soft, both physically and spiritually, keeping you flexible for the Spirit's leading. Repeat this process any time you sense that you are resisting God's direction.

Is there an area of your life where you are resisting the Holy Spirit's leading? How are you being stiff-necked?
_____
_____
_____

There is a remedy for stiff-necked syndrome, and we will explore that more during the week. For now, we can rejoice that God has provided deliverance from our pride, and that it is a free gift: Jesus Christ, His Son, our Savior. Through Him we are able to live a healthy life, free from using food as our source of comfort and finding refuge in Him alone.

Father, help me learn to bow my knee to You rather than stiffen my neck and going my own way. My stubborn pride is hard for me to relinquish, and I cannot do it without Your help. Here are the reins of my life; I choose to follow Your direction instead of my own. Amen.

—— DAY 2: SIGNS OF PRIDE
Hello, dear Father; I'm very glad to have this time with You today. Speak to my heart and refresh my spirit as I bow before You now.

One of the first steps to conquering pride is recognizing that it is normal and human. From the beginning of creation, people have resisted God's invitation to abide in His refuge and chosen instead to direct their own lives. Our pride is insidious; it keeps us from even recognizing that we have a problem with it. "I don't have a problem with pride; look how well I am doing!" It's a catch-22 situation; my pride keeps me from recognizing that I have a problem with pride.

Let's look at some religious people who were consumed by pride, people who Jesus continually confronted and condemned for their stubborn self-centeredness. Their title, Pharisee, has become synonymous with arrogance and hypocrisy. First, read Matthew 9:10-13; in verses 10-11, identify the Pharisees' complaint against Jesus.
_____
_____
_____

This characteristic of pride is *finding fault* in others. It is easy to recognize others' shortcomings while totally ignoring my own. Jesus identifies this in Matthew 7:3-5. What imagery did He use to describe a critical spirit?

_____
_____
_____

Next, let's look at the Pharisee who invited Jesus to his home for a meal in Luke 7:36-50. In verse 39, what did the Pharisee think about Jesus?

_____
_____
_____

How did Jesus reply to the Pharisee in verses 44-47?

_____
_____
_____

The Pharisee *discounted his own sin*. We may believe that we are doing fine, not sinning that much, and secure in our own righteousness. We may see ourselves as behaving better than others we know. But we are all equally in need of forgiveness, because we sin every day. Romans 3:23 says, "...all have sinned and fallen short of the glory of God." All sin comes from pride, believing I know better than God.

Another example of pride is exemplified in a story Jesus told. Read Luke 18:9-14. Describe the Pharisee in this passage.

_____
_____
_____

This manifestation of pride is *self-exaltation* and can easily affect our thoughts, feelings, and behaviors. Ironically, it can be rooted in fear of rejection or humiliation. We all need a sense of belonging and acceptance. But when we allow our anxiety over what others think about us to control us, pride becomes a false refuge.

Today we looked at three manifestations of pride: *finding fault* in others, discounting our own sin, and *exalting ourselves*. When Jesus confronted the Pharisees about their prideful ways, they went away offended and sought to remove Him from the scene. Their pride prevented them from recognizing the truth of His words. Jesus was very critical of the religious leaders of His day. They had turned God's perfect refuge for His people into a false refuge of pride for themselves. Be open to what Jesus says and the work of the Holy Spirit. He can work in you to identify and remove any pride that keeps you from true intimacy with Him.

Do you struggle with these aspects of pride? Remember pride can blind you to prideful attitudes you may have. Pride can be a cause of unhealthy eating. It can be a reason why you depend on yourself for your food choices rather than God and good nutrition facts. Carefully examine your thoughts and actions. What evidence of pride do you notice?

_____
_____
_____

Holy Father, I want to be open and honest with You and myself. Help me to truly see how fault-finding, discounting my sin, and self-exaltation may be part of my prideful ways. Let me see myself for who I truly am, so I can fully abide in You, my refuge. Amen.

—— DAY 3: THE COMPARISON CONFLICT

Today is another day to worship and praise You, Lord. During this precious time alone with You, speak to my waiting heart and show me more of Who You are.

One of my favorite childhood stories comes from the Dr. Seuss book *The Sneetches and Other Stories*. In this story, the creatures called Sneetches come in two varieties: some had stars on their bellies and some didn't. The star-bellied Sneetches thought they were better than those who had plain bellies, and they treated the plain-bellied Sneetches as outcasts. The stars on their bellies made the Sneetches proud, looking down on the others as inferior. This comparison conflict created chaos for these creatures.

For those of us who struggle with healthy choices, comparison is a losing game. We constantly look at others' bodies and think they either look better than us, resulting in shame, or that they look worse than us, resulting in pride. Both are unhealthy attitudes, no matter where we are on our wellness journey. Let's explore some of the Bible's powerful words about the comparison conflict.

Read 1 Samuel 8:1-5; what did the Israelites want and why?

God chose His people to be holy and separate from other nations in order to bring Christ into the world to redeem us all. But they wanted to be like all the other nations. What does God say about the comparison conflict in Galatians 6:4?

There will always be someone who looks better than me, at least in my eyes, and someone who looks worse. How I respond to that perception indicates my level of pride and how much it may be a false refuge in my life. We can see this truth represented in two people in the Bible: Cain and Hannah. They each faced a comparison conflict, but their reactions were different.

Read Genesis 4:1-5. Cain, Adam and Eve's firstborn son, is a farmer. In verses 3 and 5, what did Cain do and how did God respond?

Abel, the second-born, was a herdsman. In verse 4, what did he do and how did God respond?

You may have faced a situation where you felt you were treated unfairly. Perhaps you were passed over for a promotion at work, and the person who received the promotion is not the person you think is best for the job. Maybe you have sibling rivalry in your family that puts you in a secondary position that you think is unfair. Possibly someone in your circle of friends gets more attention than you, and you resent it. If so, describe your experience and how you felt.

We do not know why God accepted Abel's sacrifice and not Cain's. It could be that it was not a blood sacrifice, or that the offering was not the best of Cain's crop. Perhaps there was a difference in the attitude of each brother as he presented his offering to the Lord. What is most important is what Cain did after God's response to his offering. What warning did God give Cain in Genesis 4:6-7?

How did Cain respond to God's warning? (verse 8)

In verse 7, God said, "...sin is crouching at your door; it desires to have you, but you must rule over it." It is an interesting image of sin as a predatory animal, stealthily waiting to pounce on a sign of weakness that can lead to prideful attitudes and actions. Cain coldly murders his brother; what is his attitude about his heinous act in verse 9?

It is unlikely that Cain's callous indifference to murder developed overnight. There may have been other instances of comparison conflict with his brother before this incident. He allowed pride to rule him, and the anger he felt over God's rejection of his offering, while accepting the one from his younger brother, built up until it erupted violently. God gave Cain a chance to present an acceptable offering; Cain chose instead to kill his brother. This story shows us how pride and comparison conflicts can have tragic results, for us and others.

When has a comparison conflict caused you to be angry at another person? How did you handle it?

Hannah also experienced a comparison conflict, but she responded differently. Read 1 Samuel 1:1-8 and describe Hannah's comparison conflict.

How did Hannah handle her situation in verses 8-11?

The culture in which Hannah lived was highly critical of a woman who had no children. She faced shame and was considered sinful in some way because she was infertile. Through no fault of her own, Hannah was childless and could have been hopeless. She could have become bitter and blamed her husband or God for her situation. But she chose to take her comparison conflict to God, earnestly pouring out her heart. Rather than focusing on someone to blame, she put her trust in God. Her story ends well. Read verses 19-20 and record what happened.

We learn from Hannah that praying about a comparison conflict has much better results that acting in our own strength, as Cain did. When a comparison conflict comes my way, I can choose to take it to God rather than ignore it and let it fester inside me. Even if I don't get a happy resolution as in Hannah's case, God can change me and help me deal with my emotions in a healthy way. Are you facing a comparison conflict right now? If so, what is it?

C.S. Lewis wrote, "As long as you are proud you can't know God. A proud man is always looking down on things and people; and, of course, as long as you are looking down, you cannot see something that is above you... Pride gets no pleasure out of having something, only out of having more of it than the next man... It is the comparison that makes you proud: the pleasure of being above the rest. Once the element of competition is gone, pride is gone."[1] Checking our comparisons with others and their possessions is vital to our spiritual well-being and relationship to God and others. Jesus identified the seriousness of comparisons in Luke 18:9-14. Read this passage and summarize the Pharisee's prayer in verses 11-12.

Record this week's memory verse here.

How can you boast in the Lord today?

Father, forgive me for mishandling comparison conflicts and help me to understand the life You have uniquely designed for me to live. Remove this source of pride in me, and may I rejoice in You rather than boast in myself. Amen.

—— DAY 4: BREAKING DOWN PRIDE

My dear Father, I stop my busyness and still my mind so I can find You in the frenzy of my day. You are always with me and want to commune with me; thank You for this time alone with You.

One of the most difficult things about dealing with pride is that we are blind to it because we are proud. Here is an informal survey you may use to assess your pride level. Write beside each statement one of these letters: rarely (R), sometimes (S), or often (O).

- I am strongly defensive when someone corrects or disagrees with me. _____
- I am overly concerned about what other people think about me. _____
- I am anxious to have the last word in a conversation. _____
- I think that certain tasks are below me. _____
- I seek attention in all my social connections. _____
- I'd rather give advice than take it. _____
- In conversations, I am more focused on what I will say than I am in listening to what another person is saying. _____
- When someone is sharing a concern or asking for prayer, my first response is to tell a story about myself or share my knowledge about the same kind of situation. _____
- I talk about myself a lot. _____
- I believe my way is the best way to handle situations. _____
- I am easily offended. _____

- I do not ask for help or I believe I can take care of myself without any help. _____
- I am overly critical of others. _____
- I resist accepting other people's advice. _____
- I rationalize my mistakes and justify my sin. _____
- I want to be part of the "in crowd." _____
- I have a hard time admitting I did something wrong. _____

You likely recognized some degree of your own behavior in this list. Once we are aware of our prideful tendencies, we can take them to God for help. As we partner with Him, we can conquer it. Let's look at 2 Chronicles 7:14 for help with this process. As you read this passage, identify what God asks His people to do and the results of obeying Him.

What God Asks (4 things)	What Will Result (3 things)

On the chart, circle the first thing God asks His people to do.

Healing starts with *humility*. It is the hardest thing for the person imprisoned by pride to do. By its very nature, pride says, "I can do it myself. I've got it all figured out. I don't need anyone else's help." Admitting that this arrogant mindset is present is the opposite of pride. Look back at the survey we did at the beginning of today's lesson. Where do you see evidence of your prideful attitudes?

Read Proverbs 22:4; how does this verse define humility?

The term translated "fear" in some translations doesn't mean that I'm afraid of God as if He might hurt me. It means I have the proper respect for God; He is the Creator of the universe, the only God, omniscient, omnipresent, omnipotent, and eternal. It also means that I accept His authority in my own life. I become God-focused rather than self-focused. We are humble when we recognize our position in our relationship with God and others. Everything we have is because of God's grace, not because of our own merit. His refuge is characterized by His supremacy and my humility.

The second thing that 2 Chronicles 7:14 tells us to do is *pray*. We cannot develop humility ourselves; only pride tells us we are capable of creating our own humility. God alone can conquer pride so that we can become His humble child. The very act of prayer is bowing before God; how can we truly connect with God in prayer without humility?

Read 2 Corinthians 8:9; what is our example of humility?

_____

_____

1 Peter 5:6-7 says, "Humble yourselves, therefore, under God's mighty hand, that he may lift you up in due time. Cast all your anxiety on him because he cares for you." In order to cast our cares on Him in prayer, we must be clothed in the humility Jesus modeled.

God's third direction to His people is to *seek His face*. The Hebrew word translated "face" implies God's presence. Face-to-face interaction provides more cues to understanding what is communicated. When we seek God's face, we are looking at His character, Who He truly is. Psalm 10:4 gives us some insight into the non-example of this idea. What does it say about the wicked?

_____

_____

Andrew Murray, author of *Humility: The Journey Toward Holiness*, says, "Pride must die in you, or nothing of heaven can live in you."[2] We can look to Moses to learn more about seeking God's face. Read Exodus 34:29-35; what happened to Moses when he encountered God face-to-face?

_____
_____

What does Deuteronomy 34:10-12 say about Moses that made him unique?

_____
_____

Numbers 12:3 gives us an important clue about Moses' character; what is that?

_____
_____

We seek God's face by humbly submitting to Him and praying to Him. We don't just learn *about* Him; we *encounter* Him. Spending time in God's presence and truly seeking His face will give our lives a glow that will attract others to Him. This is our mission as kingdom people: not to call attention to ourselves, but to point others to God.

The fourth and final direction God gives us is to turn *from our wicked ways*. We cannot enter the presence of a holy God covered in sin. Confession means to agree with God that what I have done is sin. It is serious business, requiring more than just a flippant, "my bad, I'm sorry." If I agree that my actions and attitudes are sinful, then I also agree to turn my back on them and turn toward God. Turn to Psalm 66:18 and record it here. Circle the word "cherish."

_____
_____
_____

These four steps will help us leave pride's false refuge: *humility, prayer, seeking God's face,* and *turning from sin.* And we must repeat these steps many times to demolish pride; it doesn't happen overnight. But the benefits are amazing; what three things does God promise to do in the last part of 2 Chronicles 7:14? __

_____
_____

Think about areas of pride God has revealed to you. Write a prayer asking for His help in turning to Him as your refuge, thanking Him in advance for His loving power that will free you from self-centeredness, transforming you from the inside out.

_____
_____
_____

I bow before you, Lord, convicted of my prideful attitude and ways. My life is nothing without you; I can boast only in my Savior Jesus and Your salvation in me. Help me renounce my arrogance and turn away from self-centeredness, following You completely. Amen.

—— DAY 5: THREE CAUTIONARY TALES

As I come to You now, my Lord, I need to know You more. I have empty spots in my life that only You can fill. Pour Your Holy Spirit on me anew and teach me Your ways, so I may follow in them.

Learning by example is one way to learn, but learning by non-example can be more powerful. When someone makes a mistake, we see the results and know that we want to avoid that error. The Bible is loaded with non-examples, people who rejected God's perfect ways and decided they knew better. Let's explore three stories that serve as cautionary tales about how easily anyone can become prideful.

The first non-example is Moses. He was God's chosen leader of the Israelites from the Exodus through the entry into the Promised Land, over 40 years. We've already seen that he was commended for being extremely humble. But even he was guilty of pride. Read Numbers 20:2-5 and describe the situation.

_____
_____
_____

This is the third time the Bible records a similar confrontation between the Israelites and Moses. But this final time the people have been wandering in the wilderness for forty years. They refused to enter the Promised Land God had prepared for them, so they were doomed to die in the desert (Exodus 14). Now the Promised Land was in sight, and most of the generation that had rejected God's plan forty years ago had died. What happened in verses 6-8?

_____
_____
_____

How did Moses respond to God's direction (verses 9-11)?

_____
_____
_____

What was God's punishment for Moses' disobedience (verses 12-13)?

_____
_____
_____

God's response to Moses' prideful actions may seem very harsh to us. Why would God bar Moses from the Promised Land after years of faithful service because of this one act of disobedience? It must be a very serious one to have earned Moses such a severe sentence. Look closely at verse 12: "Because you did not *trust in me as holy.*" Moses ignored Who God is and took things into his own hands. Notice what Moses said in verse 10 about him and Aaron: "Must *we* bring you water out of this rock?" The people also responded to their situation with pride, forgetting that God had led them out of slavery to a better land; "Why did *you* (Moses) bring the Lord's community into this wilderness?" (verse 4) All of them forgot about the power and authority of God and acted out of their own selfish interests. Since Moses was the leader of God's people, his sin resulted in a tough punishment. If a man as humble as Moses could give in to pride, we should take heed and beware.

A second non-example of humility is a great king of Judah, Uzziah. Read Numbers 26:3-5 and describe this ruler.

_____
_____
_____

Verses 6-15 list many of Uzziah's accomplishments. List any three of them.

_____
_____
_____

Uzziah had it all: power, possessions, and popularity. He had a trusted spiritual adviser, Zechariah, who held him accountable to God (verse 5). But after Zechariah died, King Uzziah let his pride bring him down. Read verses 16-20; what did he do, and what were the results?

_____
_____
_____

Being afflicted with leprosy during this time in history was a crushing blow. Lepers had to live forever in seclusion from society, according to Mosaic Law and concerns over contagions. Describe King Uzziah's sad end (verses 21-23).

_____
_____
_____

We all need accountability; our First Place for Health group meetings and weekly contacts are critical checkpoints as we seek to develop healthy choices and love God with all our being. When Uzziah lost his accountability, he became proud. He did whatever he thought was right. We are wise if we listen to our trusted friends and those in authority over us and remain humble before God.

The third non-example of humility comes from the New Testament. On the night of the Last Supper before Jesus went to the cross, Peter acted in a prideful way. Read Mark 14:27-31. What did Jesus say all of the disciples would do on that night?

_____
_____
_____

How did Peter respond in verse 29?

_____
_____
_____

In verse 30, what did Jesus warn Peter he would do?

Peter's response is one of pride: "Even if I have to die with you, I will never disown you." (verse 31) The other disciples joined in with Peter; "And all the others said the same." Peter couldn't believe he would deny his master; he didn't stop to consider that he could be capable of this betrayal. What happened later after Jesus was arrested? Read Mark 14:66-72; what did Peter do? _

All three of these non-examples of humility before God should give us pause. These people were following God: Moses and Uzziah for decades of their lives, and Peter for three years in the very physical presence of Jesus. If these people could be swayed to respond in pride, certainly it is possible for us to do the same. What warning does 1 Corinthians 10:11-12 give us?

As you have studied these three stories, what has God revealed to you about your own pride? Spend time now in prayer with Him, asking Him to show you where you have or are likely to have a struggle with pride. Confess your prideful attitudes and actions to your loving Father, and receive His free forgiveness.

Father, You know I am prone to follow my own prideful ways rather than humbly submit to You. Why do I continue to think that I know better than You? Help me conquer my pride and find refuge in You alone. Amen.

—— DAY 6: REFLECTION AND APPLICATION

Here I am, Father, opening my mind and heart to You. I need Your strength, for I am weak, and I need Your comfort, for I am wounded. Speak to me as only You can.

I was once presented with a major change in my job that would involve me splitting my time between two departments. I immediately started mapping out a spreadsheet to organize how that would work. It involved a great deal of detail and planning out my time carefully. During this time, I was out for an early morning walk; I heard God telling me, "Today." Over and over, He impressed on me the importance of today. I realized that I was afraid of the future and wanted to avoid any problems by planning not to have them. This was not an isolated instance; it was a pattern in my life. I believed that I was the best one to plan my future, and in my pride, I was not trusting Him to handle it for me. He led me to use my daily scripture reading to help me release my pride and depend on Him, not myself, for today and the future. Since that day several years ago, almost every day, I post a scripture on my Facebook page and start it with the word, "Today." For example, "Today You, oh Lord, are my help, and in the shadow of Your wings, I will sing for joy." (Psalm 63:7) I am learning to live with God in the moment rather than seeking my own prideful plans to address my fears of the future.

Read James 4:13-16. How does this verse describe our arrogance?

_____
_____
_____

In Proverbs 6:16-19 we are given a list of seven things that God hates. What is the first thing on the list?

_____
_____
_____

What are your thoughts about leaving the false refuge of pride? What do you want God your refuge to do, and how will you participate in the process?

_____
_____
_____

Oh my God, I am ashamed of my prideful attitudes and actions. I confess that in my flesh, I want my way more than Yours. Make me mindful of my pride; help me as I let go of my selfishness and embrace You as Lord of all I am and my only refuge. Amen.

—— DAY 7: REFLECTION AND APPLICATION

How grateful I am for these daily moments with You, dear Lord. Use this time to fill me with Your Spirit and teach me in Your ways.

Use today's time with God to reflect on areas of pride He may have revealed to you. As before, you can choose how to review what God is teaching you. There have been several opportunities for journaling in this lesson, and you can go deeper on any one of them.

Optional Journaling Prompts (choose one)
- Write words and/or sketch images that represent things that build up pride in you. Then write a Bible verse that expresses your commitment to release your pride to God. An example is 1 Timothy 6:17: "Command those who are rich in this present world not to be arrogant nor to put their hope in wealth, which is so uncertain, but to put their hope in God, who richly provides us with everything for our enjoyment."
- Create or obtain an image of someone kneeling in prayer; you could have someone take a photo of you in that position. Put the image in the center of the journal page. Write a prayer around the image, confessing your pride to God and thanking Him for working in you to vacate the false refuge of pride and replace it with humility in God's refuge.
- Find a song that encourages you in this process. You may document the lyrics and record your own reflections on them, or you could illustrate them with sketches or images you locate. Two examples for this week's theme song are "Humble Heart" by Matt McChlery (2004) or the classic "When I Survey the Wondrous Cross" by Isaac Watts.

Remember to search for other's journal entries and post your own if you wish, using these hashtags on social media: #fp4h and #fp4hgodmyrefuge.

God, You know me very well, and You know my pride hinders me from knowing You more. I relinquish my hold on my pride to You now, bowing in humility before Your majesty. I am blessed that You love me in spite of my arrogance, and I thank You for the blood of Jesus that washes away my sin. I love You and want to abide in You as my only refuge. Amen.

Your Journaling

Notes
[1] C.S. Lewis, Mere Christianity (New York, NY: Macmillan, 1952).
[2] Andrew Murray, Humility: The Journey Toward Holiness, (Bloomington, MN: Bethany House Publishers, 2001).

WEEK FOUR: A REFUGE OF HEALING

SCRIPTURE MEMORY VERSE
He himself bore our sins in his body on the cross, so that we might die to sins and live for righteousness; "by his wounds you have been healed."
1 Peter 2:24

In the movie version of the book, *The Wonderful Wizard of Oz*, the protagonist Dorothy is dissatisfied with her home life. She longed to go to another "land that I've heard of." A tornado whisked her and her dog Toto off to a land full of vibrant colors and intriguing creatures, but the whole time she was there she wanted to go home. She finally got her wish, and the movie ended with the famous line, "There's no place like home!"[1]

Our God is our true refuge. Our homes and families should also be a safe refuge from the challenges and brokenness of the world. Unfortunately, that is not always the case. Some of our greatest pains may come from those who should care for us most. In the absence of a safe refuge, we may subconsciously create a false refuge to hide our pain so we can function day-to-day without being overwhelmed. But we may develop unhealthy behaviors in order to avoid the pain. For example, we might develop a pattern of emotional eating to deal with hurt or trauma.

Last week our study on God's refuge of humility focused on these concepts.
- Pride is the source of any false refuge and can cause us to have stiff necks, resistant to God's direction.
- Finding fault in others, discounting our own sin, and exalting ourselves are three sources of pride demonstrated by the Pharisees and confronted by Jesus.
- Comparing ourselves to others causes pride or shame; boast only in God.
- Breaking down the false refuge of pride begins with humility, prayer, seeking God's face, and turning from sin.
- Stories about Moses, King Uzziah, and Peter warn us to guard against pride.

This week we will look at the causes of a pain-protecting false refuge and discover healthy ways to process pain and be free. Let's pray as we begin that God will open our eyes and give us courage to face any painful truths. He is our safe place, able to heal us and restore His healthy refuge in place of the dysfunctional ones we have built.

MYplace ○ FOR BIBLE STUDY

—— DAY 1: FAMILIES THAT HURT

Thank You for today, dear Lord, for all the blessings You give me and all the people in my life. Open my eyes to Your Word now as I still myself to listen.

The Bible has many examples of dysfunctional families. Let's examine King David's parenting style. He was a man after God's own heart (Acts 13:22). He was a successful military commander and built a strong kingdom. But his parenting skills leave much to be desired. Read 1 Kings 1:5-6; what does verse 6 tell us about David's parenting style?

_____
_____
_____

Adonijah was not the only child David treated this way. What did Amnon, David's eldest son, do in 2 Samuel 13:1-2 and 10-14?

_____
_____
_____

What did Absalom do in response (verses 28-29)?

_____
_____
_____

There are no indications that David held either Amnon or Absalom accountable for their actions, except to exile Absalom for a time. He didn't intervene for his daughter Tamar. He showed favoritism to Absalom over his other sons. Absalom committed treason and stole the kingdom from David; as a result, Absalom was killed by the army. David grieved for his rebellious son to the extent that it almost turned his men against him (2 Samuel 15, 18-19).

Another dynamic of David's family can be found in 1 Chronicles 3:1-9. What was the makeup of David's family?

_____
_____
_____

David had at least eight wives; some scholars estimate he had as many as 24 wives, along with concubines. Each of the wives had sons, so it is no surprise that there was competition among David's boys. There is nothing in the Bible to indicate that David tried to manage this situation; Amnon's assault of his half-sister, Absalom's retaliatory murder of Amnon, followed by his treason are dramatic examples of how David failed as a father. He was responsible for the dysfunctional dynamics of his family.

Deuteronomy 17:17 says, "[The king] must not take many wives, or his heart will be led astray." David did not heed this command in the law, and his family became a hotbed of dysfunction. Perhaps you experienced dysfunction in your family of origin or in the family you have as an adult. Parenting that is too lax or too strict can hurt children in various ways. Paul also warns against this problem in Ephesians 6:4; what does he say about parenting?

_____
_____
_____

Some families have Christ at the center, and some do not. What does Paul warn us about in 2 Corinthians 6:14?

_____
_____
_____

There are many types of dysfunctional families; here are five kinds:
- Substance abuse
- Conflict-driven
- Violent
- Authoritarian
- Emotionally detached2

What are some ways your family of origin impacted your life, both in healthy and hurtful ways?

_____
_____
_____

In response to these fractured family dynamics, children often subconsciously develop internal walls to shelter the pain and cope with life. They may use self-destructive behaviors to keep the walls strong and avoid dealing with the hurt. Substance abuse, including eating too much or too little food, is a common practice. If you excessively use food for comfort or suffer from an eating disorder, you may have built a false refuge to contain pain. That is how I coped with the family pain I experienced.

How do we begin to replace a false refuge and enter instead into God's perfect refuge? It can be a long, difficult process. In my own life, it took many years to work through the pains I experienced in my home. Although my parents were loving and wanted what was best for me, they were human and made mistakes. God has been with me and given me strength and hope throughout the process. Here are some things that are helpful for me.

- **Saturate yourself with God and His Word** – I learned to read at an early age, and I began reading the Bible often. I listen to songs that have scripture lyrics. Filling myself with God's Word gives me direction and hope. What does Hebrews 4:12 say about the power of God's Word? __
- **Confide in trusted friends** – God sent key people into my life to help me cope with my emotional hurts. I have two friends I met in 7th grade who I still talk with regularly; I can and do tell them anything, and they are always there for me, even though we don't live in the same community. If you are a trusted friend, learn to listen well. Your prayers, comfort, and honesty are vital to your friend's healing. How does Proverbs 18:24 describe this kind of friend? __
- **Seek Christian counseling when needed** – Throughout my adult life, there were times when the process of dealing with the pain was more than I could handle on my own. Several Christian counselors have helped me through those times. What direction do we read in Proverbs 13:10 about wise counsel? __
- **Commit to the hard work** – I will not sugar-coat the experience of healing from family fractures. It is some of the most difficult work I've done. I have wept, written in my journal, spent sleepless nights praying, and felt confused and in despair. But God never abandoned me, and He continues to help me. It has been a process for me, and when I had a breakthrough, the freedom was sweet. What does Philippians 2:12-13 tell us about this process? __

In his book *You Will Get Through This*, Max Lucado reminds us that Jesus is our big brother. We all come from a dysfunctional family: the human family. Each one of us has rejected our Father through pride, rebellion, and sin. Our brother Jesus died for us before we even knew Him.³ He will help you with your emotional pain and free you. What is a first step you can take this week to begin or continue that process?

_____
_____
_____

What is the main thing holding you back from taking this step?

_____
_____
_____

Have faith in the One Who created you and loves you beyond belief. He is with you, dear friend, and He will never leave you because He is your true refuge.

Dear Father, I have experienced pain in family relationships. Please help me to recognize a self-created refuge and allow You to work in me to remove it. Use Your Word and Your people to guide me along the way. I commit to the process of healing and trust You to do it. Amen.

—— DAY 2: GRIEF AND LOSS

Holy God, thank You for opening Your throne room to me today. It is only through the blessed Name of Jesus my Lord, Who has given me life through His blood, that I can boldly enter into Your presence. Speak to my heart and change me as we meet now.

Another source of pain comes from grief and loss. Let's explore two examples in scripture. The first story is about Naomi and Ruth; what happened to them in Ruth 1:3-4?

_____
_____
_____

Naomi lived in a foreign land when this happened. She returned to her home in Bethlehem, and people were surprised to see her with only her daughter-in-law. What was Naomi's response in Ruth 1:20-21?

_____
_____
_____

Ruth was from Moab, a nation that had been in conflict with Israel for years. Naomi encouraged Ruth to stay in Moab when she was leaving to go home. What was her response (verses 16-18)?

_____
_____
_____

Both women experienced great loss. Naomi lost all three members of her family; Ruth lost her husband and gave up her homeland. Life for widows in their patriarchal cultures was extremely difficult. If you had no sons to provide for you, you had to get by the best you could. There was no government welfare or charitable organizations to help you. Naomi was too old to earn a living doing manual labor, and Ruth was an immigrant from a despised neighboring country. Their situation was dire. As often happens for those of us who have lost a husband, the emotional grief is compounded by financial difficulty.

The second story about grief we will examine is the parable about the prodigal son. Luke 15:11-16 tells us about the younger of two sons in a family. As you read these verses, consider the father's perspective and imagine how he felt. What did the son do?

_____
_____
_____

Now read verses 17-24, continuing to focus on the father's experience. What did the son decide to do, and how was he received?

_____
_____
_____

Have you waited for family members to "come to their senses?" It is a long and heart-wrenching process to watch someone you love choose to reject God and follow a self-destructive path. Notice that the father let the son go; he didn't try to enable him or make excuses for him. He sent him on his way and waited for him to come home. Not every story of waiting for a prodigal to return has a happy ending like this one. The grief and loss of a wayward person can be as overwhelming as that of a loved one's death.

Finally, let's read verses 25-32. There is another person in this story that brings grief to the heart of the father. What was the prodigal son's brother's reaction to his return?

_____
_____
_____

It's interesting that this story is commonly titled "The Prodigal Son;" however, Jesus actually told this story to point out the attitude of the son who stayed home. He was confronting the Pharisees who complained that Jesus was ministering to "tax collectors and sinners" (Luke 15:1-2). He wanted them to see how their relationships to the Father were self-centered and sinful, based on what they could do to be superior. They judged those who were not like them, and they criticized Jesus for caring about them. They were prodigals, too. These self-righteous religious leaders did not see themselves as members of the same family as the "tax collectors and sinners," family members who should care for each other. Perhaps you have experienced a family conflict where there is anger, hurt, and estrangement between two or more people. The grief and loss is compounded when the situation goes on for a long time.

When we experience grief and loss, we are in excruciating pain, a normal and healthy reaction. However, we must be careful to properly process our pain so that the pain doesn't get trapped within a false refuge, festering and poisoning our beings. Holding on to the pain doesn't help the situation change or help us become whole. Letting go is hard and scary, but it is the only way to healing. What does Paul tell us in Philippians 4:6-7?

_____
_____
_____

The prayer Paul talks about here is profound. It is not a flippant, "Help me, Lord," kind of prayer. It is the falling on your face, pouring out your soul, screaming and sobbing, and pounding your fists kind of prayer. And it isn't a one-time event; the Greek syntax implies persistence in the prayer. Continue to *pray until the peace comes*. And don't miss the hope in the passage: "with thanksgiving." We are not thanking Him *because* we are in pain; we are thanking Him that *He is with us* in the pain. God understands pain from death and loss; His prized creation, humanity, has been prodigal since the beginning. He allowed His only Son to experience pain, injustice, and death. Whatever you are feeling, God understands. What does Hebrews 4:14-18 say about His ability to empathize with us?

_____
_____
_____

Sweet friend, if you are in the midst of grieving, be comforted by God and your trusted friends. If you have unresolved grief, be brave and bring it to Him. Keep working through the pain; there are better days ahead. God will walk with you every step if you will follow His lead. Allow Him to remove the barriers that keep you from facing your pain and grief so that He can bring healing to your soul and surround you with His true refuge. I've experienced it many times, and His refuge is faithful and true.

My Father, I lay my needs before You now; You know the depths of my pain and grief. Whatever the source, You are my hope. Help me work through this pain with You, as long as it takes, as deep as I must go. I confess I can be whole only when I let it go. Thank You that You are with me through it all. I love You. Amen.

—— DAY 3: TREATING TRAUMA

Hello, dear Father. I'm glad You are here to meet with me now, to show Yourself to me in new and meaningful ways as I study Your Word. Give me eyes to see and ears to hear.

Another source of pain that can result in a false refuge is trauma. Trauma comes from physical or emotional injury. It can happen in stressful situations of varying magnitudes, such as fighting in a war, being in a wreck, or suffering abuse. It can be from one major incident or a combination of several events. The psychological response to the pain of the incident is trauma, and the symptoms, ranging from mild to severe, may either be immediately identified or show up much later. The effects can be healed easily and quickly or can have long term implications. A person may develop Post-Traumatic Stress Disorder (PTSD) if the symptoms persist and are not resolved. One response to this pain is to build a false refuge to cope with it. A temporary defense mechanism may become permanent, leaving the pain from the trauma unresolved.

Although almost everyone experiences trauma to some degree in one form or another during their lifetimes, a smaller percentage develop long-lasting effects that require treatment for healing. But everyone who experiences trauma needs love and support. Whether you are looking for that comfort or you are one who gives comfort to a trauma survivor, our true refuge is found in a loving God.

Earlier this week we evaluated King David for his poor parenting skills. Let's revisit his life and see how he encountered and handled trauma. Read 1 Samuel 20:1; what was David's situation at this time?

_____
_____
_____

He fled King Saul's court; where did he go (1 Samuel 21:10)?

_____
_____
_____

Gath is a significant place for David, for the giant Goliath he killed came from there. He must have been desperate to escape King Saul to go there. What happened in King Achish's court (verses 11-13)?

_____
_____
_____

King Achish sent David away; David's ruse worked. Later David wrote a psalm of thanksgiving for God's redemption from this traumatic event. Read Psalm 34, keeping David's story in mind, and focusing on verses 18-19. How does David describe God's care for those who experience trauma in these two verses?

_____
_____
_____

We can be assured that the help we need is in the Lord. That is the spiritual side of healing from trauma; there is also a physical aspect. When we experience trauma, it affects our brains. The area that involves thinking and reasoning along with the center of emotion are under activated, but the part of our brain that deals with fear is over activated. "If you are traumatized, you may experience chronic stress, vigilance, fear, and irritation. You may also have a hard time feeling safe, calming down, or sleeping. ...You may notice difficulties with concentration and attention ...can't think clearly [or] feel incapable of managing your emotions."[4] This physiology emphasizes the connections between the physical and emotional parts of our beings and helps us understand how trauma affects our thoughts, emotions, and behaviors.

There are several things ways to deal with trauma as you engage God in the healing process. The first step is recognizing that trauma happened and affects you. Healing never begins until the source of trauma is brought into the light. What promise do you have in Psalm 145:18?

_____
_____
_____

Facing past pains can be scary. Depending on the length of time since the traumatic event and the strength of the false refuge, it may require intense treatment. You can be confident of God's abiding presence; what promise is in Isaiah 41:10?

_____
_____
_____

Next you can pray for God to reveal the false refuge. How did you build it and keep it strong? It is usually a behavior that is self-destructive, sometimes secret. For many of us, it is emotional eating. In prayer, tell God about your pain and your false refuge. Hiding our pain only makes it worse. What does Psalm 32:3-7 say about bringing our brokenness to God for healing?

_____
_____
_____

Notice that the psalmist is open about his pain; God can only heal what we honestly feel. The road to recovery from trauma begins with a small step and is followed by a multitude of small steps. It is rare that someone recovers with a single dramatic episode; more likely it happens with daily practices that culminate in wholeness. I have dealt with trauma; as a child I believed I had to be strong for my family when my parents separated, and I was mocked for years because I was overweight, by my father and classmates. I went through a divorce then the death of my ex-husband. I can testify that God my refuge was with me every step of the way; I was never closer to Him than during the hard work of recovery and healing.

Let's finish today's study with verses from God's Word that became a vital part of my healing process. Read these words from Joel 2:25-26.

> "I will repay you for the years the locusts have eaten—
> the great locust and the young locust,
> the other locusts and the locust swarm—
> my great army that I sent among you.
> You will have plenty to eat, until you are full,
> and you will praise the name of the Lord your God,
> who has worked wonders for you;
> never again will my people be shamed."

God spoke through this passage when I was going through healing from trauma, and I clung to His promise of restoration. He has surely kept His promise, healing me and giving me new life and hope. I am deeply grateful to my loving Father and His persistent patience in my life. He is my refuge.

Thank You, Father, for being with me through this process of restoration. I am unable to tackle the pain alone, and I am grateful for Your constant presence. Give me strength and hope as I face the hard work of healing, knowing You will repay me for the years that the locusts have eaten. I trust You. Amen.

—— DAY 4: BOUNDARIES, NOT A FALSE REFUGE

Dear Lord, this is the day You have made, and I choose to rejoice and be glad in it. My heart is open to Your leading; speak to me now.

Butterflies are lovely. They are colorful, symmetrical, and airy. It's hard to believe that such beauty starts out as an ordinary grub. Butterflies go through a process to become what they were created to be. They form a cocoon and after a while, they break through the cocoon, changed from an earth-bound worm to an airborne wonder. It struggles as it emerges from its shell. If you were watching, you might think you could help it by breaking the casing to release it. But you would actually be damaging it, because it is through the work of cracking the cocoon that the butterfly becomes strong enough to fly. If it doesn't do the work itself, it will be weak and deformed.

We may respond to pain by becoming fixers, like trying to help the butterfly rather than letting it struggle. In 1 Samuel 2:12-17 and 22, we meet a man who did this with his sons. What did the Israelite priest Eli's sons do in their tabernacle service?

_____

_____

_____

How did Eli respond to his sons' actions, and what effect did his response have on them (verses 22-25)?

_____
_____
_____

In 1 Samuel 2:27-29 Eli is confronted by a man of God; describe why God is upset with Eli.

_____
_____
_____

"…you honor your sons more than Me." Eli didn't hold his sons accountable for their sin. He even participated by eating the parts of the offering that were meant for God. When the man of God says "[you are] fattening yourselves on the choice parts of every offering made by my people Israel (verse 29)," he meant it literally. 1 Samuel 4:18 tells us that Eli was "heavy," meaning overweight. Eli didn't take action against his sons' disobedience. His false refuge of pride kept him from dealing with his sons appropriately.

As we tear down a false refuge, we may find that we have not set healthy boundaries in our relationships. It is difficult to watch someone struggle with pain and grief, and we can be supportive and caring. But we can't fix other people. In her book Surrendered, Barb Roose puts it this way: "I am not in control of others or outcomes."[5] Instead of building a false refuge to protect ourselves from dealing with pain and trauma, we can instead spend our energy on building healthy boundaries that give us space and keep us from interfering in others' lives. Think about boundaries as fences between neighbors. It doesn't mean you don't care about your neighbors if you have fences around your yard. The fences define the limits of what belongs to you and what belongs to them. It keeps you from constantly fighting over where your property lines lie. The same is true with personal boundaries; you establish them to ensure you are free to work on your life while others work on theirs.

God set the first boundary in the Bible in Genesis 2:15-17; what limit did he put in the Garden of Eden?

_____
_____

Why did He establish this limit (verse 17)?

___

Read Galatians 6:2-5. In verse 2, what are we told to do?

___

What is the balance in verse 5?

___

These two statements may seem contradictory: do we carry another's burden or our own? It is a balancing act for us as Christians to help each other without doing all the work for people who need to do the work for themselves. We must all process our own struggles to grow, to become the butterflies God created us to be, while supporting each other in healthy ways.

Setting proper relationship boundaries is critical to good mental health. Here are some suggestions.

- **Learn to *say no*.** Suppose someone where you work is constantly asking you for help so that you end up doing some of that person's work along with your own. The next time the person asks you for help, you can say no. You could word your response something like this: "My plate is full right now; I have to focus on my work." Saying no is an important part of setting healthy boundaries. Saying no is not un-Christian. Jesus said no at times. He regularly set aside time to be alone and pray (Luke 5:16). He didn't go to heal Lazarus before he died (John 11:6). Setting boundaries is not selfish; it is self-care.
- **Rework your understanding of *responsibility*.** If you are over involved in another person's life, or you allow others to be over involved in your life, personal responsibility has been hijacked. Consider how you are responsible for your own thoughts and actions; let go of controlling the other person's decision-making power. And if you have allowed someone to commandeer your choices, begin

taking back control of your own life. God created each of us as individuals, unique and special, to have individual lives and relationships with Him.
- **Focus on what is true.** If you are in an abusive relationship, do not believe the lies that say you are the problem. If you have loved ones who abuse substances, do not believe the lies that say you are responsible for their choices and can fix them. Do not make excuses for them. Do not try to protect them from the consequences of their actions. The most loving thing you may do is set the boundaries for healthy relationships which benefit both of you. God's Word is truth, and immersing yourself in it every day will help you see your life and others' lives more clearly. Ask God to give you His vision about your relationships and His help to see and accept the truth.

A school principal shared a story with me about interviewing prospective teachers. One candidate was chosen for the job, and letters were sent to the others who had applied. Soon afterwards, a woman came to the school and asked to see the principal. The woman was the mother of one of the people who were not hired, and she wanted to find out why her daughter didn't get the job. This type of helicopter parenting is an example of poor boundaries in relationships. It is likely a result of the mother's pride and fear, a false refuge that not only damaged her life but intruded on her daughter's life as well. Do you have problems with boundaries in any of your relationships? If so, what are they?

Let us pray for God our refuge to show us how healthy boundaries can keep us focused on Him and what He wants to do in each of our lives. Let's become the beautiful butterflies He created us to be, made in His image and involved in the process of becoming like our blessed Savior, Jesus Christ.

Almighty God, You are the source of all truth and You know me better than I know myself. Help me to clearly see the boundaries in my relationships. Give me courage to take action when my boundaries are not healthy and clearly defined. Thank You for Your love and strength. Amen.

—— DAY 5: THE GIFT OF PAIN

Today I praise You, Lord, exalting Your Name for all You are and do. I thank You that You hear me as I speak to You now, and I wait quietly to listen to Your voice.

Hansen's disease is a bacterial infection that affects a person's nerves, respiratory system, eyes, and skin. During Biblical times, people who contracted it were called lepers. They were outcasts who lived in colonies away from the general population, because the disease was considered highly contagious. One of the difficulties of leprosy is that the nerve endings in some parts of the body don't work. For example, lepers are prone to developing blindness, because they don't blink their eyes when needed. They can't feel irritation that can harm the eyes. *The Gift of Pain* is a book based on Dr. Paul Brand's lifelong work in treating patients with Hansen's disease; his co-author Phillip Yancey gave this viewpoint about pain.

> Pain is not something that most of us would count as a blessing. However, Dr. Paul Brand's work with leprosy patients in India and the United States convinced him that pain truly is one of God's great gifts to us. In this account of his fifty-year career as a healer, Dr. Brand probes the mystery of pain and reveals its importance. As an indicator that lets us know something is wrong, pain has a value that becomes clearest in its absence. Indeed, pain is a gift that none of us want and yet none of us can do without.[6]

Our pains can be used by God to change us. It is human nature to avoid pain at all costs. That's why we may retreat to a false refuge: to avoid the hurt we fear. God our refuge has the balm that will heal our pain, but we have to bring the pain to Him to experience healing. Let's explore some Bible verses that can help us be transparent about our pain with our loving Father.

Let's start with our memory verse, 1 Peter 2:24. Write it here, practicing your memorization of the verse.

_____
_____
_____

What do you notice about the source of our healing?

_____
_____
_____

Paradoxes are prevalent in the Bible: we die to live, we humble ourselves to be exalted, and we give to receive. Peter quoted from an Old Testament verse (Isaiah 53:5) that contains another paradox. Jesus' pain brings us healing. He knows what pain is all about, because He experienced it Himself, more deeply than we ever will.

There are several benefits from truly experiencing pain. First, pain is a warning system. When we feel pain, we know something isn't right. Most people resist going to the dentist. But if you have a toothache, you will likely overcome that resistance and make an appointment to find out why your tooth hurts and have it fixed. If you had no pain, your tooth would continue to deteriorate until it was beyond help. Read Psalm 119:71-72; how do these verses relate to the importance of pain as a warning system?

_____

_____

_____

Another advantage of feeling pain is that is *cultivates character*. The story of the Velveteen Rabbit explains this concept well. The rabbit was a new toy in the nursery and was initially overlooked as its owner favored trucks and building blocks. As it sat sadly with the other neglected toys, the Skin Horse had a conversation with him. The rabbit wondered if he would ever become a real rabbit, not just a stuffed toy. The Skin Horse said, "Real isn't how you are made. It's a thing that happens to you. When a child loves you for a long, long time, not just to play with, but REALLY loves you, then you become Real... Generally, by the time you are Real, most of your hair has been loved off, and your eyes drop out and you get loose in the joints and very shabby. But these things don't matter at all, because once you are Real you can't be ugly..."[7] God's love for us allows us to experience pain so we can become the authentic persons He created each of us to be. Pain hones us, removing the rough parts and revealing the genuine beauty beneath.

Job certainly understood this process; what does he say in Job 23:10?

_____

_____

_____

Romans 5:3-5 has a list of benefits we receive when we are going through difficulties. List the benefits here.

_____

_____

_____

What does James 1:2-4 encourage us to consider?

What is the ultimate benefit of experiencing pain here on earth? Find the answer in 1 Peter 4:6-7.

It is not easy to accept pain as a gift when you are in the midst of it, and that is okay. Pain can develop perspective that allows you to see your life from God's viewpoint. Healthy healing from pain doesn't require a "pull yourself up by your bootstraps" mentality. It is about honestly opening your heart to God so He can bring the healing. But understanding that pain can have an eternal purpose in your life to help leave a false refuge behind.

Dr. Paul Brand spent his life working with people suffering from Hansen's disease. He saw first-hand its terrible effects on thousands of patients. He was asked if he would eliminate pain, if he could. He responded, "If I held in my hands the power to eliminate physical pain from the world, I would not exercise it… Thank God for inventing pain."8 May we also learn to thank God in our pain and depend on Him for healing and wholeness. It truly is "a gift that none of us want and yet none of us can do without."

Oh, dear God, You know the depths of my pain. You understand my resistance to facing it. But I know You are with me, holding me in Your loving arms. Help me to accept the healing You provide and the perspective I need to see pain as a gift. Amen.

—— DAY 6: REFLECTION AND APPLICATION

I'm glad to meet with You today, Lord. My every desire is known to You as I come into Your presence now. I put my hope in You, Lord, and I know You will respond to my desires as I open my heart to You.

During some of the counseling I have experienced, I was encouraged to create a safe place in my mind. It is a place that I could run to when I felt overwhelmed as I processed my feelings. I imagined a beautiful beach with crystal blue water, a lounge chair under a palm tree, and a sunny day with a bit of breeze. I named the place "Peaceful Blue." Retreating to this peaceful mental scene was healthier for me than using food to comfort myself. Eating our pain doesn't deal with the pain but temporarily soothes it. Then we are left with more weight and a less healthy body. Removing a false refuge takes times and persistence, and there are times you may need to step away from the work and rest in the safety of God's refuge.

Do you believe God is a safe place for you to bring your pain? Why or why not?
___
___
___

Read the following verses, and record how each one gives you hope for healing from pain in the protected refuge of God.

Verse	Hope for Healing from Pain
Psalm 30:1-2	
Psalm 103:1-3	
Isaiah 41:10	
Isaiah 58:8-9	
Jeremiah 17:14	
Ephesians 3:20-21	
Revelation 21:3-4	

Consider creating a mental safe place. You can even designate a literal place in your home that you can go to when you are meeting with God to process your thoughts and feelings. If you were to create that space for yourself, what would you call it, and what would it look like?

___

Write a prayer to God your refuge about where you are in your process of dealing with pain. You might express your concerns about facing your pain, what you think about Him being a safe refuge for you to bring your pain, or thank Him for what He has or is doing to help you with your pain. Be honest with Him; He is trustworthy. Use your journal if you need more room to write.

___

Lord, I anchor my soul in Your haven of rest, where I find healing, peace, and love. My life is in Your hands, and my being is in Your keeping, for You are the source of all life and my deliverance. I rest in You for all I need; thank You for soothing my pain and embracing me with Your strong, safe arms. Amen.

—— DAY 7: REFLECTION AND APPLICATION

Holy God, as I come before You today, I anticipate a time of sweet fellowship and encouragement. Give me wisdom as I seek You and understanding as I hear what You have prepared for me.

This week may have been intense for you as you have considered past pains and fractured family relationships. Wherever you are with these issues, God is with you. Imagine His arms encircling you as He tells you how much He loves you, you are His special child, and He will always be your refuge. For your reflection time today, you may choose to review some of the personal questions and responses you recorded in this week's study.

Optional Journaling Prompts (choose one)
- Write a goodbye letter (not to send) to the person or persons who caused you pain. Say everything you wanted to say when you were hurt but probably didn't

say. Be honest with how it felt and how it has affected you. Once you have finished, write a prayer thanking God that this pain no longer has any control over you. Ask Him to help you let it go and leave it with Him. If you feel the pain coming back, return to this journal entry and remind yourself that you have let it go and said goodbye. It may take many times before you notice a change, but you are making a positive step toward healing.
- Find a video or series of images of a butterfly shedding its cocoon. Imagine yourself doing the same thing with your pain, fighting to open up the outer shell and becoming stronger as you break free. Record how that feels and thank God for His deliverance from the cocoon caused by your pain.
- Locate photos of your family of origin or current family. Include a copy of the photos in your journal. As you study your family members' faces, write your feelings, both positive and negative, about how each impacted your life. Be honest and pay attention to anything that needs prayer and healing. What would you want a photo of your family to look like after God has brought restoration?
- If you have created a mental or physical safe place, locate images that represent what that space looks like to you. If it is an actual place, take a picture of it. Put the images in your journal, and write about why these images make you feel safe. You can add scripture verses, such as Isaiah 26:3: "You will keep in perfect peace all who trust in you, all whose thoughts are fixed on you!" (The New Living Translation)
- Find a song that encourages you in this process. You may document the lyrics and record your own reflections on them, or you could illustrate them with sketches or images you locate. Two examples for this week's theme song are "Healer" by Hillsong (2008) and "You Are My Hiding Place" by Ledner Michael James (1981).

Remember to search for other's journal entries and post your own if you wish, using these hashtags on social media: #fp4h and #fp4hgodmyrefuge.

I bring all I am to You, Father, knowing You are my only hope of healing and wholeness. All I am and all I have is from You, and I want to become free from anything that keeps me from knowing You completely. Thank You for helping me process the pains in my life so I can be free indeed. I love You. Amen.

Your Journaling

---

[1] Victor Fleming, et. al., The Wizard of Oz (Metro Goldwyn Mayer: 1939).
[2] Amen Clinics, "Which of the 5 Types of Dysfunctional Families Do You Have?" 2020. https://www.amenclinics.com/blog/which-of-the-5-types-of-dysfunctional-families-do-you-have/.
[3] Max Lucado, You'll Get Through This (Nashville, TN: Thomas Nelson, 2013).
[4] Jennifer Sweeton, "How to Heal the Traumatized Brain," March 13, 2017, Psychology Today. https://www.psychologytoday.com/us/blog/workings-well-being/201703/how-heal-the-traumatized-brain.
[5] Barbara Roose, Surrendered: Letting Go & Living Like Jesus. (Nashville, TN: Abingdon Women, 2020).
[6] Phillip Yancey, "The Gift of Pain," 2021. https://philipyancey.com/books/the-gift-of-pain.
[7] Margery Williams Bianco, The Velveteen Rabbit: or How Toys Become Real (New York, NY: Doubleday, 1922) 5-8.
[8] Paul Brand & Phillip Yancey, The Gift of Pain (Grand Rapids, MI: Zondervan, 1997).

WEEK FIVE: A REFUGE OF MERCY

SCRIPTURE MEMORY VERSE
The Lord is gracious and full of compassion, slow to anger and great in mercy. The Lord is good to all, and His tender mercies are over all His works. Psalm 145:8-9

A story is told about the nineteenth century French emperor Napoleon. A mother once approached Napoleon seeking a pardon for her son. The emperor replied that the young man had committed a certain offense twice, and justice demanded death. "But I don't ask for justice," the mother explained. "I plead for mercy." "But your son does not deserve mercy," Napoleon replied. "Sir," the woman cried, "it would not be mercy if he deserved it, and mercy is all I ask for." "Well, then," the emperor said, "I will have mercy." And he spared the woman's son.

I have discovered in many years of working on my own fitness journey along with leading dozens of First Place for Health groups that we are incredibly hard on ourselves. We can be our own worst critics and tormentors when it comes to making healthy choices and our weight. We rarely offer ourselves mercy but hear instead an internal voice of condemnation. Do you have an inner critic? Stacy Julian, a creative innovator, writer, and podcaster, gave her inner critic a name, Persephone, so that she could better identify, quiet, and manage the constant heckling in her head.[1]

Last week in "God My Refuge," we considered these truths about healing.
- Dysfunctional families can be a source of deep pain, but God our Father and Christ our brother love us and can heal us.
- When we experience loss and grief, God is in the pain with us.
- God can bring healing to trauma and its effects on our lives.
- Healthy boundaries are necessary for healed relationships.
- Pain is a gift, serving as a warning system and character cultivator.

This week we will explore God's refuge of mercy and how basking in that mercy can heal our wounds and satisfy our souls. We can quiet our inner critics by saturating our minds with the truth of God's unlimited love and.

—— DAY 1: WHAT IS MERCY?
Today is a new day, God, a day full of Your blessings and wonders. Open my eyes to see all You have prepared for me to experience today, and quicken my heart to seek

WEEK FIVE   A REFUGE OF MERCY

Let's start our study this week with an understanding of Biblical mercy. Look up the word mercy in a dictionary and record your findings here.

_____
_____
_____

Now check a thesaurus and choose three words that you think best describes mercy as you understand it.

_____
_____

In the Bible, the word translated "mercy" comes from two words: *checed*, a Hebrew word which has the sense of goodness, kindness, and faithfulness; and *eleos*, a Greek word which denotes kindness or good will towards the miserable and the afflicted, joined with a desire to help them.[2] Imagine you see someone on the street who clearly needs help. They may have tattered clothes, dirty skin, and unkempt hair. The feeling of compassion you may have is not really mercy, however. Mercy is taking the person to a restaurant and buying a meal to feed him. Mercy is action, not emotion.

Read Luke 6:32-36. How does Jesus describe mercy?

_____
_____
_____

There's an important characteristic of God in these verses: "He is kind to the ungrateful and wicked." That goes beyond feeling compassion for someone who is in need; that is giving up my right to judge someone who I feel doesn't deserve my help. It may even be someone who wronged me. That is generosity beyond human capacity. That is not giving what is deserved but giving what is undeserved.

Write this week's memory verse here.

_____
_____
_____

When was the last time you experienced mercy from someone other than God?

_____
_____
_____

When was the last time you offered mercy to someone?

_____
_____
_____

How merciful are you? Put a check beside any of the actions below that you believe you are very likely to do.

_____ When someone I know is recuperating from surgery, I send a card, visit, and/or take food to that person.

_____ When a person in my life who rubs me the wrong way offends me, I am quick to forgive, whether or not she asks for forgiveness.

_____ When I see people in need who I don't know, I stop to help them in some way.

_____ I intentionally look for ways to help people rather than wait for an opportunity to fall in my lap.

_____ When I make a mistake on my food plan, I forgive myself and try again without condemning myself.

It is easier to offer mercy to those in our inner circles. But if we start to look beyond our own walls, if we encounter those who are different from us in culture or political persuasion, if we look at our own mistakes – those situations may be more difficult for us to respond mercifully. How can we learn to practice mercy as God our refuge does? That will be our goal this week as we study God's refuge of mercy.

_____
_____
_____

God, help me to understand Your mercy. You have freely given it to me, and I am deeply grateful. Show me when and how to offer mercy to others and to myself in ways that honor You. I love You, Lord. Amen.

—— DAY 2: GOD'S MERCY TOWARD YOU
Thank You for another day to live for You, my Father. How good it is to praise You and worship You with all that I am. Speak to me now as I study Your Word and sit in Your presence.

The Bible has several themes that run through it; one of those themes is God's mercy. Over and over again, God provides mercy when He could mete out punishment. Examine these examples.

Genesis 3: How did God show mercy to Adam and Eve? (verse 21)

This act is significant; what does Hebrews 9:22 tell us about what God did?

Genesis 4: How did God react with mercy to Cain after he murdered his brother? (verses 10-15)

David was called "a man after God's own heart." (1 Samuel 13:14) What characteristics do you think qualifies him for this moniker?

What were David's sins chronicled in 2 Samuel 11?

What were the consequences of his sin? (2 Samuel 12:11-14)

How did God show David mercy (verse 13)?

Later God offered an additional act of mercy toward David in 2 Samuel 12:24-25. Record the amazing gift David received.

_____
_____
_____

Even a sin as great as David's was not beyond the mercy of God. Perhaps you think his sins were too heinous for God's mercy. Maybe you believe justice would have been a better response from God in this situation. I'm glad that God gets to make those decisions instead of me. His mercy is greater than mine, and He is able to balance mercy and justice with His great wisdom in ways that are beyond my understanding.

These are some examples of how God showed mercy to people in the Bible. But what about you? How has God shown you mercy? Let's check out these passages. Record your thoughts about God's mercy beside each one and consider how He has shown you mercy?

Psalm 25:10

_____
_____
_____

Psalm 145:8-9 (this week's memory verse)

_____
_____
_____

Micah 7:18

_____
_____
_____

The phrase "...but God" is powerful. I'm grateful that my life didn't end with my evaluation of myself. Before I joined First Place in 1981, I was full of self-loathing for being overweight and in despair that I would never get better. "But God" had other plans for me, and His plans were full of mercy. I didn't deserve His help to overcome my failures with weight loss and healthy boundaries in my life. My efforts were feeble and futile. "But God" offered me mercy; He took me and transformed me. He continues to give me mercy every day, because I still struggle to totally obey Him.

How amazing that He offers the same mercy to every single person who has ever lived, is living, or will live on Earth. No matter where you are in your faith journey and your fitness progress, you can depend on God for mercy that covers all your sin. Let's thank Him for His unending mercy toward us!

Lord, thank You for Your great mercy toward me. I do not deserve Your compassionate care for me, yet You offer it to me anyway. I'm grateful for my life as You have created and planned it for my best and Your glory. Help me to see Your mercy and accept what You offer me. Amen.

—— DAY 3: MERCY TOWARD YOURSELF

Father, I am in need of Your presence. I know that it is the only place where I can find refuge. As I meet with You now, fill my being with Your Spirit, reveal my innermost thoughts, and change me.

Paul was a mighty man of God. He preached the gospel everywhere he went, and he desired deeply to follow God completely. Surely there have been few people who followed God as closely as he did once he accepted Christ's call. But he was still human, and he confessed his struggle with sin. Read Romans 7:13-25 and summarize Paul's dilemma.

_____
_____
_____

Paul found that knowing the law was not enough to free him from sin. Perhaps you have discovered that knowing how to make healthy food and exercise choices hasn't been enough for you to live outside a false refuge that causes you to be overweight and unhealthy. Just learning about the food plan hasn't made you change your behavior. Perhaps you can relate to Paul's struggle; I know I can!

Thank God Paul doesn't stop here. We have already looked at Romans 8:1-2; let's review what it says in light of Paul's struggle in Romans 7:13-25. What is God's response to Paul's situation?

_____
_____
_____

God's response toward your failure to live up to perfection is mercy. He does not give you the sentence you deserve. He offers mercy every time you rebel against His best plan for you. He offers mercy when you turn away from Him in your time of need and choose another way to soothe yourself. He never gets tired of offering mercy to you, and He never runs out of mercy. His supply is endless.

Why is God able to provide mercy? Read Titus 3:5 for an answer.

Christian comedian and musician Mark Lowry tells a story about getting up very early one morning. His alarm clock rang loudly at 4:30 a.m., and he struggled to get out of bed. He stubbed his toe walking in the dark of the pre-dawn hours. He said, "I did not feel saved. I did not look saved. I did not smell saved. But if Jesus comes again at 4:30 in the morning, I'm going!"[3] His point is that our relationship with God is not based on our feelings or appearance. If you feel condemned, it is not coming from God. When you sin, He doesn't condemn you if you have accepted Jesus' gift of salvation. The condemnation you feel is coming from your inner critic or the enemy. We can choose whether or not to believe a verdict of condemnation.

Our sin may have consequences, just as Adam, Eve, Cain, and David experienced. We can choose to confess our sins, repent, and receive forgiveness (1 John 1:9). And we may continue to struggle with sin and repeatedly ask God for forgiveness and help to overcome it. But condemnation is never a part of the equation if you are in Christ Jesus. He took on our punishment for sin to make God's mercy possible.

If you haven't yet received this gift of mercy, you can do that now. Jesus has provided a way for you to have access to God even though you are not perfect. You can pray to Him and ask Him for His merciful forgiveness and begin a new life, free from the burden of condemnation. You can know the assurance and peace that only He can give you. If you want help with this decision, ask your leader for assistance.

Do you struggle with self-condemnation? If so, what is keeping you from offering mercy to yourself?

Look again at Romans 8:1-2. Rewrite the verses here and substitute your name in this way: "Therefore, there is now no condemnation for *Debbie* who is in Christ Jesus, because through Christ Jesus the law of the Spirit who gives *Debbie* life has set *Debbie* free from the law of sin and death." __

Now read that text aloud, emphasizing your name and "Christ Jesus." Read it again and emphasize "no" and "free." Do you believe it? Say it again until it is real to you. Make it a daily confession if you find you need to hear it again. You are free from condemnation! God's refuge is full of mercy because Jesus has paid the price for us.

Thank You, Father, for Your mercy toward me. I believe in the freedom You have provided to me through Christ Jesus my Lord. Help me to reject condemnation from the world, from the enemy, and from myself, and instead embrace the liberty of walking in the Spirit. Amen.

—— DAY 4: YOUR MERCY TOWARD OTHERS

As I come into Your presence now, I am thankful for Your love and mercy. I need it again today and every day. Open my heart to Your voice and Your Word.

When we see someone who breaks the law or hurts other people, we can be quick to judge and demand restitution and punishment. And justice is important; God is a just God. But He is also merciful, and He calls us to extend mercy to others in the same way. God describes Himself in Exodus 34:6-7, which this week's memory verse references. Read the verses and record the attributes of God's mercy you find in them.

The Jews list 13 different attributes of God's mercy in this passage from their Talmud. As you read these attributes, identify three words or phrases that resonate most with you and circle them.

1. The Lord! (*Adonai*)–God is merciful before a person sins! Even though aware that future evil lies dormant within him.

2. The Lord! (*Adonai*) – God is merciful after the sinner has gone astray.
3. God (*El*) – a name that denotes power as ruler over nature and humankind, indicating that God's mercy sometimes surpasses even the degree indicated by this name.
4. Compassionate (*rahum*) – God is filled with loving sympathy for human frailty, does not put people into situations of extreme temptation, and eases the punishment of the guilty.
5. Gracious (*v'hanun*) – God shows mercy even to those who do not deserve it, consoling the afflicted and raising up the oppressed.
6. Slow to anger (*ereh apayim*) – God gives the sinner ample time to reflect, improve, and repent.
7. Abundant in Kindness (*v'rav hesed*) – God is kind toward those who lack personal merits, providing more gifts and blessings than they deserve; if one's personal behavior is evenly balanced between virtue and sin, God tips the scales of justice toward the good.
8. Truth (*v'emet*) – God never reneges on His word to reward those who serve Him.
9. Preserver of kindness for thousands of generations (*notzeir hesed la-alafim*) – God remembers the deeds of the righteous for the benefit of their less virtuous generations of offspring.
10. Forgiver of iniquity (*nosei avon*) – God forgives intentional sin resulting from an evil disposition, as long as the sinner repents.
11. Forgiver of willful sin (*pesha*) – God allows even those who commit a sin with the malicious intent of rebelling against and angering Him the opportunity to repent.
12. Forgiver of error (*v'hata'ah*) – God forgives a sin committed out of carelessness, thoughtlessness, or apathy.
13. Who cleanses (*v'nakeh*) – God is merciful, gracious, and forgiving, wiping away the sins of those who truly repent; however, if one does not repent, God does not cleanse.[4]

God's mercy is deep and wide, beyond our ability to understand. Yet as His children who reflect His image and character, we are called to be merciful as well. Instead of desiring revenge in our humanness, God wants us to act with mercy. Read Matthew 5:44; what did Jesus command His disciples to do?

_____

_____

_____

In our relationships with others, the way that we offer mercy is important. Consider the difference between sympathy and empathy.

- Empathy: feeling with someone, focus on the one in pain, get in the feelings with her
- Sympathy: feeling for someone, focus on your feelings, impose pity on her

Most of the time we are likely feeling sorry *for* someone rather than feeling *with* that person. When we extend mercy and feel sorry for someone, it might be less comforting for that person. The listener says these things because he is uncomfortable with and not sure how to respond to the person in pain. The hurting person needs to hear that she is loved and not alone, not what the listener needs to say to help him deal with her pain. Here are four things that we might do that disrespect the person's pain and put the focus on us instead.

- **Bright-sider:** say something positive no matter how bad the person hurts
  "At least your cancer is treatable!"
- **It's-not-so-bad-er:** minimize her situation
  "It's not so bad for you because…"
- **Fix-er:** try to fix her problem with advice or solutions, even when he is not an expert in the field
  "You should do this because I've read an article about…"
- **Let-me-tell-you-bout-er:** tell stories about self or others who have had similar circumstances, especially how others have had it worse
  "When I went through this experience, I did this…"[5]

Here's an example of a "let-me-tell-you-bout-er." I contracted a serious case of shingles a few years ago. I was in unrelenting, excruciating pain for three months. One of my friends heard about my suffering and told me about someone who had shingles and suffered pain for years. Although factual, I didn't need to hear that! In the midst of my pain, I needed comfort and hope, not the worst-case scenario. Why did my friend say that to me? Like most of us, she believed she was commiserating with me and meant well. But she was *sympathizing*, not *empathizing*.

God's empathy for us is great. Read Psalm 56:8 in the New Living Translation; how personally does He participate in your pain?

Isaiah 53:4-5 relates what Jesus did for us; read these verses and reflect on what His sacrifice means to you.

His mercy is beyond our understanding and compels us to give mercy to others as we have received it from Him. God is merciful; being merciful to others is reflecting the image of God. Is there someone in your life to whom you need to extend empathy today? If so, who is it and what can you do?

_____
_____
_____

Father, people all around me every day are in desperate need of Your mercy. Please give me the will and the strength to respond with empathy and not sympathy, just as You have extended empathy to me. Amen.

—— DAY 5: GRACE: THE OTHER PART OF MERCY

How blessed I am to be Your child, dear Lord. Your mercies are new every morning; great is Your faithfulness. I am ready to hear Your voice right now.

We have looked at mercy, which is not giving someone the punishment they deserve for bad behavior. God's character also includes the flip side of this coin: grace. The Bible dictionary describes grace as "the unmerited favor of God toward man. In the Old Testament, the term that most often is translated 'grace,' is hen; in the New Testament, it is charis."[6] Therefore, mercy is not receiving the punishment you do deserve, whereas grace is receiving good you don't deserve.

We saw mercy first illustrated in Genesis 3 after the fall of humanity. Grace appears for the first time in Genesis 6. Read verses 9-14; what did God tell Noah He would do and why?

_____
_____
_____

What did God offer Noah and his family to save them from destruction?

_____
_____
_____

Romans 3:24 tells us how all people experience salvation: "...and all are justified freely by His _____ through the redemption that came by _____ _____."

WEEK FIVE A REFUGE OF MERCY

Noah may have followed God more closely that those who lived during his time, but he didn't earn the right to ride out the storm on the ark. He and his family were saved by God's grace. God gave him something he had not earned.

Just as experiencing God's mercy helps us develop a merciful attitude and behavior, experiencing God's grace encourages us to be gracious. We can learn to give good to ourselves and others whether or not we feel it has been earned.

There is an interesting story in Jeremiah 52. King Jehoiachin was a wicked king of Judah. 2 Kings 24:9 tells us that "he did evil in the eyes of the Lord, just as his father had done." He and his entire family was taken away in chains to Babylon. His throne was given to his uncle. While King Nebuchadnezzar ruled, Jehoiachin remained imprisoned. Imagine Jehoiachin's surprise when one day, after 36 years in captivity, the prison door opened. Light streamed into the dark chamber. He heard the clank of metal and felt chains fall off his wrists and ankles. The jailer took him out of the cell where he had been trapped for such a long time. He was given a bath, and his beard was trimmed. He dressed in clean clothes and new sandals. He was led into the presence of the king. He learned that King Nebuchadnezzar had died and his son was now in charge. Read Jeremiah 52:31-34; what gracious act did King Awel-Marduk offer Jehoiachin?

_____

_____

_____

Jehoiachin had done nothing to deserve his freedom and the honors he received. He had no resources to offer in exchange. Only his captor's grace gave Jehoiachin a new life. The name of King Awel-Marduk is translated "Evil-merodach," not a person from whom you would expect to receive grace. "But God" (There it is again!) was able to work through a pagan king to offer grace to Jehoiachin.

You were imprisoned as well, taken captive by sin and locked away for life. "But God" has removed your chains. He has freed you from your food addiction, your unhealthy choices, and your rebellious spirit. What do you have to do to live daily in that freedom? What did Jehoiachin do in verse 33?

_____

_____

_____

What does "putting aside [your] prison clothes" mean to you?

_____
_____
_____

Perhaps you are in need of a dose of grace. Your fitness journey may be long and hard, and you may experience bumps along the way. You may still struggle with food choices, exercise routines, or spiritual disciplines. Please know that God is right there with you, offering you "grace upon grace" (John 1:16, ESV). Your hard work and devotion to His plan for you will pay off, because He is a gracious God, giving you far more than you deserve.

Thank You for Your amazing grace, Father. You have given me much more than I deserve. Help me to put aside my prison clothes and walk in the freedom that You offer me through Jesus my dear Savior. Amen.

—— DAY 6: REFLECTION AND APPLICATION
Thank You for meeting me with now, Father God, and fill me with Your Spirit. I have needs that only You can fill, and I'm trusting You now for all that I need.

Today we will consider our inner critic, the one who constantly tells us how bad we are, how we've messed up, and how we can't possibly deserve anything good in our lives. What words or images come to mind when you are critical of yourself?

_____
_____
_____

Why do you believe you think these critical thoughts?

_____
_____
_____

You are worthy of God's love, mercy, and grace – not because you've earned it but because He has declared you worthy. You are so worthy of good from God that He sent His Son to save you from this type of inner critic language, from any condemnation. As you reflect today on God's mercy, consider the ways He has made you who you are today, "gracefully broken but beautifully standing."[7] Thank Him for the many ways He has cared for you throughout your life. You may want to write in your journal about one or more of those instances of His mercy and grace to you.

_____

_____

_____

Finish today's reflection by meditating on 1 Peter 1:3-4; record it here.

_____

_____

_____

Father, I am thankful for Your refuge of mercy, for Your protection, and the way You use even difficult times in my life to mold me into the image of Your Son, Jesus. Thank You that I am gracefully broken but beautifully standing. Amen.

—— DAY 7: REFLECTION AND APPLICATION

I find my hope and joy in You alone, O Lord. Use this quiet time with You to transform me into the person You created me to be. I'm listening and excited about what You will say.

A young woman was traveling by stagecoach, reading a book. One phrase struck her as particularly meaningful. She was so entranced with the words she turned to a man sitting next to her and shared them: "Prone to wander, Lord, I feel it; prone to leave the God I love." As she talked about the words, the man began to weep profusely. He said, "Madam, I am the poor unhappy man who wrote that hymn many years ago, and I would give a thousand worlds, if I could enjoy the feelings I had then." Robert Robinson was indeed the author of the hymn "Come Thou Fount of Many Blessings." But since writing the song, he had turned his back on God. The woman reminded Robinson of the other words he had written in the hymn: "Streams of mercy, never ceasing." It's unclear whether or not Robinson came back to God, but His mercy was available to him nonetheless[7]

God our refuge offers mercy beyond measure. We cannot sail beyond the oceans of mercy He has for us. We need that mercy daily in light of our struggles with sin and life in a broken world. Take time to reflect on His mercy in your life.

Optional Journaling Prompts (choose one)
- As you read the Bible daily, record instances of God's mercy. What can you learn from these examples, and how can you use them to inspire you to respond in mercy to yourself and others?
- Record ways that other people offer mercy to you. Consider thanking them in person or in writing for their acts of mercy.
- Find images that reflect the idea of mercy and put them in your journal. They can be actions of people or images that symbolically represent mercy. Write captions or descriptions for each image.
- Pray that God will show you how to practice mercy. Keep a list of your own acts of mercy, and thank Him for giving you the opportunity to show His mercy to others.
- Consider people in your life who need mercy from you. How will you respond in mercy to these people? Pray God will lead you to practice mercy in His power and in His Spirit.
- Find a song that encourages you in this process. You may document the lyrics and record your own reflections on them, or you could illustrate them with sketches or images you locate. Two examples for this week's theme song are "The Mercy Seat" by Don Moen (2000) or "Mercy" by Matt Redman (2013).

Thank You for the seat of mercy that You provide, dear Lord. May I be constantly in Your presence and humbly receive Your mercy. Change me, Father, so I may become like Jesus. Amen.

Notes

1 Stacy Julian, "Exactly Enough Time, Episode 2: Distracted & Questions," February 7, 2019. https://www.stacyjulian.com/podcast/episode-2-distracted-amp-questions.

2 Bible Study Tools: Mercy, 1996. https://www.biblestudytools.com/dictionary/mercy/.

3 Mark Lowry, "Mark Lowry: My First Comedy Video," (Nashville, TN: Word Music, 1988).

4 Ronald L. Eisenberg, "The 13 Attributes of God's Mercy." https://www.myjewishlearning.com/article/the-13-attributes-of-mercy/.

5 Carlos Whittaker, "Human Hope" podcast, That Sounds Fun Network, episode 2, 2020. https://podcasts.apple.com/us/podcast/episode-002-can-empathy-heal-racism-sexism-all-bad/id1249486443?i=1000512533128.

6 Bible Study Tools: Grace, 1996. https://www.biblestudytools.com/dictionary/grace/.

7 Attributed to Denis Darothchetche, source unknown.

8 Kenneth W. Osbeck, 101 Hymn Stories: The Inspiring True Stories Behind 101 Favorite Hymns (Grand Rapids, MI: Kregel Publications, 2012) 52.

Your Journaling

WEEK SIX: A REFUGE OF FORGIVENESS

SCRIPTURE MEMORY VERSE
The Lord is good, a refuge in times of trouble. He cares for those who trust in him. Nahum 1:7

In Shakespeare's play Hamlet, Prince Hamlet discovered that his uncle killed his father. He became obsessed with revenge for his father's death. By the end of play, Hamlet exacted his retribution by killing his uncle, but he and six other people close to him died as well. An invading army occupied his country, and only one friend was left to tell his sad story. His revenge was extremely costly.

When we are hurt, it is natural to be angry at the one who caused us pain. It is normal to have feelings of revenge. But obsessing over or enacting revenge only exacerbates the pain; it doesn't erase it. Anger and revenge may turn into a false refuge of bitterness.

Last week we examined God's mercy and the refuge it provides.
- Mercy is not receiving the bad things we deserve.
- God offers mercy in unending supply to everyone.
- God doesn't condemn us but provides freedom in Christ. We can choose to give ourselves mercy rather than self-condemnation when we fail.
- As we have received mercy from God, we are to extend mercy to others; empathy is a better way to communicate caring than sympathy.
- Grace is receiving something good we don't deserve. God graciously gives us freedom in Christ, so we can put aside our prison clothes with which sin has enveloped us.

This week we will consider God's refuge of forgiveness and the dangers of bitterness and vengefulness. There are other ways to respond to those who hurt us. Jesus has the answer for our pain; through His love, we can embrace forgiveness and the freedom that it brings.

—— DAY 1: BITTER WATER

You are my King, oh Lord; You ordain my victories. I boast in You all day long and praise Your Name continually. Speak to me now as I bow in Your presence.

Water is one of life's essentials. We can survive without water for only a few days. Today we can choose from a variety of versions: filtrated, artisanal, flavored, and carbonated. In some places in the world, getting water every day is a struggle. One may have to go for miles to collect and carry water for drinking and home use.

Water is a repeated image throughout the Bible. It is in the Garden of Eden (Genesis 2:10), the flood of Noah (Genesis 7), and deliverance of the Israelites from the Egyptians (Exodus 14). Once the Israelites left the Red Sea and were on their way to the Promised Land, they discovered that there was no potable water in the wilderness. Read Exodus 15:22-24. What was the problem, and how did they respond?

_____

_____

_____

What did they call the place and why?

_____

_____

_____

This scene is repeated throughout decades of wilderness wanderings. The Israelites faced a crisis, they complained about it and blamed God, and Moses provided a solution through God's direction. We looked at some examples earlier in this study. When Moses gave his farewell address before they entered the Promised Land, he warned the people about the consequences of their idolatry. Read Deuteronomy 29:16-18. What is the warning?

_____

_____

_____

For what two reasons did God make His covenant with Israel?

_____

_____

_____

The "bitter and poisonous fruit" is connected to the rebellion at Marah. The people didn't trust God to provide for them, even after He had repeatedly shown Himself to be faithful. They praised God and sang to Him at the beginning of Exodus 15 for His miraculous power over the waters of the sea. But a few days later they didn't trust Him to provide water in the wilderness; how ironic. How easy for us to criticize them, and how easy for us to do the same thing: lose faith in God when our throats are parched and all we can see is bitter water in front of us. The bitterness is about their rebellion more than it is about the taste of the water.

Water can become bitter when it isn't pure. It may have salt, sediment, or pollutants in it. And our lives can become bitter when we allow the desire for revenge to settle in our hearts. This bitterness is rooted in unforgiveness, one source of a false refuge introduced in Week 2. Let's expand our understanding of unforgiveness and its relation to bitterness.

Previously we studied God's refuge of healing from pain and trauma. When pain is not processed in a healthy way, it can fester, leading to resentment, anger, and depression. In an effort to relieve the pain, we may turn our attention to the one who hurt us. Whether or not the hurt was intentional, the perpetrator becomes our target. We want that person to hurt, too. We want revenge. We may even seek to bring about revenge to some degree. It is normal to experience this initially, but if we let the thoughts and feelings take up residence in our being, they can hurt us even more than the original pain.

The solution to our desire for revenge is forgiveness with God's help. Depending on the depth of your pain, it may be a long process. But forgiveness produces amazing healing and freedom. This week we will find ways to seek forgiveness that will bring release. For today, let's end our time in God's Word with His assurances that He loves and cares for us. Read the following verses and record how God's love and power impacts you.

John 16:33

_____
_____
_____

Ephesians 3:17-19

_____
_____
_____

Romans 5:6-8

As you reflect on God's love for you, open your heart to His healing power and retreat to Him as your refuge. What are your thoughts at this point about dealing with bitterness?

Dear Jesus, You are the source of living water, the water that can refresh and clean me, the water I desperately need. Show me where I am holding on to bitterness or unforgiveness, and help me release those attitudes to You. I want to be full of You, not my hurt and anger. Give me Your peace. Amen.

—— DAY 2: UNRESOLVED ANGER
My loving Lord, I praise You for You are the one true God Who fights for me. You have given me Your best – Your beloved Son – and I am grateful for Your precious forgiveness. Speak to me now as I seek You.

What makes you angry? Perhaps it's getting cut off in traffic. Maybe you become angry when someone in your life doesn't live up to your expectations. Or your source of anger may come from abuse or mistreatment by someone you trusted. When someone hurts us, it is normal to feel anger and to feel the perpetrator should pay. Those feelings are not sin. What does Ephesians 4:26-27 say about this anger we feel?

Verse 26 is a reference to Psalm 4:4 in the Septuagint (the Greek translation of the Old Testament). It says "…in your anger, do not sin." The anger is not the sin; it is our response to anger that can lead to sin. The phrase, "Don't let the sun go down on your anger," is not literal in meaning. But it does imply urgency; anger needs to be dealt with quickly. If it is left to its own devices, it takes root in our minds and hearts.

The false refuge of bitterness is related to others we've examined, including pride and jealousy. Consider this metaphor: "Bitterness is unforgiveness fermented."[1]

Something that is fermented sits for a long time and chemically develops into a new substance. Grapes are fermented into wine by adding yeast to its juices and controlling temperature and oxygen levels. Good wine is created when the liquid is carefully fed and nurtured. In the same way, anger develops into bitterness when we nurture it and let it grow.

Let's return to Naomi in the book of Ruth. Did she have reason to be angry? Of course. She was living during a famine and had lost her husband and two sons in a foreign land. Read Ruth 1:20-21; what did she say about herself when she returned home?

_____
_____
_____

The word "Mara" is the same word used in Exodus 15 when the Israelites encountered bitter water. They blamed God for bringing them into the desert, although He had rescued them from the Egyptians. Who is Naomi blaming?

_____
_____
_____

We have a choice when it comes to how we respond to hurt and pain. Once again, it is normal to lash out and want to blame others and God. But if we stay stuck in that mindset, we can't find healing and peace. Fortunately for Naomi, she didn't stay stuck in her anger. First, she didn't deny her anger and pain. She was honest about her feelings; pretending we are not angry or hiding it only delays healing. Next, rather than stew over her loss, Naomi redirected her attention. Read through Ruth 2; what became her new focus?

_____
_____
_____

Her daughter-in-law Ruth had also suffered loss. But she didn't sit around and dwell on it; she found a new purpose – caring for her mother-in-law Naomi. And Naomi found new purpose in encouraging and advising Ruth.

Sometimes our anger can come from jealousy. In Week 3 we looked at the comparison conflict in relationship to pride. That jealousy can also feed anger if we refuse to process it and let it go. Read Psalm 73:1-5 and summarize the psalmist's feelings.

_____
_____
_____

It is easy to maximize our own pain and suffering because it is close to our minds and hearts, and at the same time minimize the problems others face. And when the person who hurt us goes unpunished and appears to have no problems, we may feel like the psalmist in verse 13: "Surely in vain I have kept my heart pure and have washed my hands in innocence." But as the psalmist pours out his heart to God, he chooses to change his thinking. Read verses 23-28; on what does he focus in this part of the psalm?

_____
_____
_____

One thing I notice is that the psalmist began to see his relationship to God as more important than his righteous anger. And the ending is key – he still believed the wicked should be punished, but he left it to God. He realized that God would deal with them in His time and His way. This step is vital in healing from pain and releasing anger. Until I resign my self-appointed position as judge and jury over the ones who have hurt me, I will continue to struggle with anger and bitterness.

How do you respond to angry feelings? Do you have unresolved anger or hold grudges against anyone?

_____
_____
_____

Consider the analogy of fermenting wine. As long as you feed your anger and deny it the exposure it needs to heal and release, you will continue to develop bitterness. That bitterness hurts you, not the person who offended you. And bitterness can interfere with your relationships, thereby hurting others. Pray for guidance in dealing with any unresolved anger so you may fully abide in God's refuge of forgiveness.

Lord, I do not want to develop bitterness in my heart. Sometimes it is hard to let go of anger, because I have been hurt deeply. I need You to help me release these feelings of anger and revenge. Replace them with Your love and peace, and remove any trace of bitterness from me. Amen.

—— DAY 3: BLAME GAME

How wonderful to be with You today, dear Lord. Talking to You and studying Your Word is my nourishment. Open my heart to Your Spirit's work during this quiet time with You.

Yesterday we looked at the Israelites and Naomi and times when they blamed God for their difficult situations. When we are angry, when we are hurting, we normally look for someone or something to blame. But playing the blame game can strengthen a false refuge of bitterness. Let's compare two people in the Bible who reacted differently when they were confronted with their sinful actions. First, let's read about King Saul in 1 Samuel 15. He did not follow God's directions about fighting against the Amalekites (verses 1-3). When the prophet Samuel confronted King Saul about his disobedience, what excuse did he give (verse 24)?

_____
_____
_____

Playing the blame game meant King Saul took the focus off his own disobedience and shifted it to his men. This incident is not the only time King Saul played the blame game. He became a very bitter man, blaming David for his problems and seeking to kill him. When David became king, he was confronted by a prophet about his own sinful acts. Read 2 Samuel 12:7-10 and summarize what David had done.

_____
_____
_____

How did David respond in verse 13?

_____
_____
_____

Notice David didn't make any excuses or shift blame. David recorded his prayer to God in response to this event in Psalm 51. Read verses 3-4; what do you notice about his prayer?

_____
_____
_____

King Saul fell into the blame game that seeks to shift responsibility for one's actions to someone or something else. King David did not; he immediately accepted his culpability for his crimes with no excuses or blame. He suffered consequences for his sin, but his relationship to God was restored.

Why do we play the blame game? One answer is pride, a common source for a false refuge. Another reason is fear. We are afraid of guilt and shame. We are afraid of being wrong. We are afraid of dealing with the consequences of our mistakes. Read James 3:13-14; what do these verses say about humility, bitterness, and honesty?

What if you have been wronged, and it truly is someone else's fault? What if you have been abused? It is important to know that the abuse is not your fault. Holding yourself responsible for abuse you experienced is on the other end of the blame spectrum and is dishonest. However, if we blame the offender for poor choices we make as a result of his mistreatment, we perpetuate the pain and it won't heal properly.

In Romans 8, Paul talked about troubles we have in life and God's care for us in all of them. After he listed some of these troubles, he anticipated several questions his readers might ask in response. He started Romans 8:31 with "these things," referring to the troubles he listed. As you read Romans 8:31-39, record his answers to these questions.

"What, then, shall we say in response to these things?" (verses 31-32)

"Who will bring any charge against those whom God has chosen?" (verse 33)

"Who then is the one who condemns?" (verse 34)

"Who shall separate us from the love of Christ?" (verses 35-39)

_____
_____
_____

Verse 37 is a key part of Paul's Romans 8 treatise: "In all these things, we are more than conquerors through Him Who loved us." Write your name in the blanks below and read this statement aloud several times, emphasizing different words in the sentence. Think about the meaning of these words: *You are a victor, not a victim.*

In all these things, _____ is more than a conqueror through Jesus Who loves _____.

Victims are helpless, victors are not. We can reject fear of guilt and shame. If you are blaming yourself for what your abuser did to you, please hear these truths. If you are blaming another and ignoring your responsibility for a mistake you made, please hear these truths. God has provided forgiveness and healing; we do not have to assign blame to settle the score. He has taken care of it all through Jesus' death on the cross. Release the blame and accept His righteousness. He took on all the blame for us so we can live as victors. Deal with your sin as David did by coming clean and knowing that God your refuge will continue to love you. Confidence in His love and forgiveness will help us stop playing the blame game.

Are you playing the blame game? Who or what do you blame for not meeting your fitness goals? What steps do you need to take to be honest and stop blaming?

_____
_____
_____

Father, create in me a clean heart; renew a right spirit within me. Restore the joy of my salvation, the forgiveness from my sins. Help me to stop blaming others when I am wrong. Help me to stop blaming myself when I am not wrong. And help me to trust You and Your Word, which says I am a conqueror, not condemned. Amen.

—— DAY 4: AUTHENTIC FORGIVENESS

My loving Lord, I praise You for Your great power and wisdom. As I step into the light of Your presence, I seek to know You more. Prepare me for the words You have ready for me.

When God established His covenant with the Israelites on Mount Sinai, He gave them rituals and laws so that they could develop godly habits and stay in right relationship with Him. Their faith in Him would be evident in their obedience to His covenant terms. Exodus, Leviticus, and Numbers give the details of these 613 specific directions. However, by the time Jesus began His ministry the list had expanded to thousands of rules and regulations. In Matthew 23:23-24; what was Jesus' condemnation of these leaders?

_____
_____
_____

The Jews put conditions on God's original perfect covenant. He wanted contrite hearts, not code conformists. As we approach the practice of forgiveness, we must evaluate the condition of our hearts. Forgiveness is not easy or natural but a divine response to human offense. It is the solution to bitterness and choosing to become better instead. But we must understand that we cannot do it ourselves, and we must understand that it takes *practice*.

How easy or hard is it for you to forgive someone who has hurt you?

_____
_____
_____

It is vital that we develop a Biblical understanding of forgiveness. The first example of forgiveness in the Bible is in Genesis 3. Read through verses 8-24 and look for the place where Adam and Eve asked for God's forgiveness. Record it here.

_____
_____
_____

Did you have trouble finding it? Yes, because it isn't there. God forgave Adam and Eve, but *they didn't ask for forgiveness*. There is no record of their confession of their sin or a request for absolution, only blame for each other, the snake, and even God (verses 12-13). But He provided them with forgiveness along with the consequences of their sin. God showed us what forgiveness looks like from the very beginning of creation.
- He didn't wait for a request for forgiveness before providing it. In fact, He had it ready since He knew they would sin before they did. He has an eternal heart of love and forgiveness for all humanity.
- He didn't protect them from their sins' consequences. He was still their Father, but they suffered exile and hardships because they chose their way rather than His.

- He didn't stop loving them and pursuing relationships with them. God doesn't exit the story in Genesis 3. He is on every page of the Bible, continually seeking restoration with His creation. He outlined His redemptive plan in Genesis 3:15: "And I will put enmity between you [the serpent] and the woman, and between your offspring and hers; he will crush your head, and you will strike his heel." From the beginning, God planned to provide ultimate forgiveness through His Son Jesus, born of a virgin, Who died on the cross to defeat the enemy, sin, and death.

What does that mean for us as we practice forgiveness like God? First, we must confront the offense. Don't make excuses for what happened or try to rationalize the reasons. Just name it and feel it. Read Matthew 5:21-24. In verses 21-22, Jesus warned us about what?

_____
_____
_____

He gives us an example of what this looks like in verses 23-24. What does He instruct us to do concerning forgiveness?

_____
_____
_____

Asking for forgiveness and offering forgiveness is part of a faith walk with Jesus. But it begins with recognizing that an offense has taken place. In verses 23-24 Jesus gives us the next step: *confront the offender/offended.* Talk to the person and seek reconciliation. What if the person doesn't respond or is unreachable? You can still offer or receive forgiveness. I had an experience where I needed to forgive some people who had hurt me deeply. Confronting them in real life was not the best solution, so God led me to do it in a different way. I found a picture of them and put it in a chair. I sat opposite the chair, looking at the picture. Then I poured out my heart to them, speaking out loud, about all the times they had hurt me, whether or not they meant it. I cannot put into words the freedom I felt once I had finished. My face was tear-stained, and my voice was hoarse after talking for almost an hour. As I released my pain and anger and began to forgive them, I left the false refuge of bitterness behind.

If you have been abused, it may not be healthy or possible for you to confront your abuser. We looked at healthy boundaries previously; it is important to set them for protection. But you can still confront your abuser in an alternative way as I did. It may take more than one attempt to completely be free of anger and bitterness. It requires God's help, because forgiveness is not easy for us.

Third, we must release the revenge. The one who has offended you may have to face consequences for his hurtful behavior. It may mean you must back off from your relationship with him and maintain healthy boundaries. Don't allow anyone to continue to abuse you; that is not good for you or him. Forgiveness doesn't mean the person you are forgiving is off the hook for the consequences of their behavior. It's just not up to you to enact the punishment. That's God's role.

Read Romans 12:14-21; what do you think it means in verse 12 to "bless" those who persecute you?

That's a radical idea: bless someone who persecutes you! Speaking words of blessing over an enemy seems like a crazy way to live, but Jesus modeled it for us. He forgave those who crucified Him, right on the spot (Luke 23:34). We all need forgiveness just as those who hurt us do.

In verses 15-16, what are we instructed to do?

We might call this response *empathy*, which we looked at last week. It is recognizing others' feelings and being supportive with the focus on them, not us. We are asked to do the same thing with those who persecute us. It is easy to rejoice when they suffer something; it's like we're getting even with them. My friend Helen Burgess speaks truth when she says that we want justice for others but mercy for ourselves! But as Christians we are called to empathize with everyone, not just those who are our friends. Notice that means we have to relinquish our pride.

Romans 12:17-21 challenges us to treat our enemies differently than we would like to treat them. Summarize these verses.

Is there a specific situation to which you could apply these verses? What can you do to practice this type of behavior?

What does 1 John 4:19-21 tell us about loving others?

One key to loving others who hurt you is focusing on the love God lavishes on you and His constant supply of forgiveness for your offenses toward Him. Release the need for revenge to Him; then you can be free from bitterness.

We can practice forgiveness with these actions.
- Confront the offense
- Confront the offender/offended
- Release the desire for revenge

These practices give us power to vacate a false refuge of bitterness and become better as we choose God's refuge of forgiveness. It is worth the intention, repetition, and work of God's Spirit to live a life free from bitterness. What can you do in the next few days to begin or continue to practice forgiveness?

Forgiveness is a tough ask, God. I have pains that are hard to heal and the need for revenge is strong. I need You and the power of Your Spirit in me to work on this challenge. Show me my next step, and help me take it in faith, knowing Your forgiveness of my sins is always available to me. Amen.

—— DAY 5: LETTING GO FOR GOOD
As I meet with You now, Lord, I am trusting You to show me where I am holding on to my anger and sense of justice for myself and others. I know You have a better way to replace my bitter way; please help me give my bitterness to You.

These past four days' lessons have detailed a process that is hard but worth it. Stay with it today and in days to come when bitterness may threaten to develop. Practice choosing God's better way. Write this week's memory verse here.

_____

_____

_____

We can choose to let go of our bitterness because of God's faithfulness and care for us. We can trust that when we let go of anger, He will fill us with His healing and love. Consider what it looks like to live without bitterness. Jesus gave us examples in Matthew 5-7. His Sermon on the Mount gives many instructions for how to live a life apart from a false refuge of bitterness. We'll look at a few examples here, but you may want to read through all three chapters later, focusing on how Jesus instructs His followers to live with love instead of anger.

Matthew 5:2-12 are referred to as the Beatitudes, meaning blessings. The idea of being blessed in the Bible includes the idea that we reach the full potential God created us to be. Jesus didn't identify separate groups of believers in these verses. Rather He detailed characteristics that all His followers display or are developing as they follow Him. The Beatitudes are a portrait of people who are better, not bitter. List the believers' characteristic and blessing Jesus gives us in each of the following verses from Matthew 5.

Verse	Characteristic	Blessing
3		
4		
5		
6		
7		
8		
9		

Verse	Characteristic	Blessing
10		
11-12		

Which characteristic is most important to you as you think about living without bitterness? Why?

_____
_____
_____

Jesus fleshes out the ways His kingdom people live without bitterness in the rest of the Sermon on the Mount. Let's consider some illustrations that He gives us and identify the attitudes and behaviors they represent. The first one is given as an example.

Verses	Kingdom People's Attitudes and Behaviors
5:21-22	Let go of anger.
5:38-42	
5:43-48	
6:1-4	
6:19-21	
6:25-34	

How do you think that these attitudes and behaviors reflect a life free from bitterness?

_____
_____
_____

One note of clarification: Jesus is not describing His followers as doormats. Rather He is describing how kingdom people live in a fallen world. We develop strong character and increasing dependence on Him as we encounter persecution. We leave the need for revenge to Him and focus on loving others as He loves us. Loving others includes not allowing others to abuse us or violate healthy boundaries. It does not include compromising the truth; Jesus never did. Kingdom people are strong, not weak, because they put their trust in God, not in themselves, others, or this world's systems.

Another aspect of eliminating bitterness concerns community. God created us for relationship, both with Him and others. His kingdom is filled with people relating to each other, not living in isolation. One of the best parts of belonging to a First Place for Health group is the bond we share. We meet regularly and talk personally about how God is working in our lives to develop all four parts of our beings. I cannot imagine following God in this way on my own. I need my Christian family to love, support, and challenge me on this journey. Read Hebrews 12:14-15; what description is given here of a healthy Christian community, and how is it a way to prevent a false refuge of bitterness from growing?

_____
_____
_____

You may notice that grace is the opposite of bitterness. It is a way to protect me from a false refuge. Look up Ephesians 4:31-32; what does Paul tell us to do instead of becoming bitter?

_____
_____
_____

"Forgive just as Christ has forgiven you." Here is where I can let go of anger and bitterness for good. Focusing on what God has done for me through Christ, Who chose to forgive me before I even knew I needed His forgiveness, sacrificed Himself through death on the cross, rose again to conquer sin and death for me, and helps me let go of the pain others cause me. His grace and mercy pale in comparison to my anger and bitterness. I must practice letting go, but I will never let go if I don't practice. Continue to develop a mindset of forgiveness and grace as you walk in the Spirit and seek God as your refuge rather than clinging to anger and bitterness.

God, help me desire Your blessings more than I desire to cling to my bitterness. Help me to trust You, focusing on the redeeming love You offer me through Christ. Empower me through Your Spirit to release my anger and bitterness. I want to be better, not bitter. Amen.

DAY 6: REFLECTION AND APPLICATION

Holy Father, I desire to abide in Your presence today. I am quieting my spirit and mind so I can hear You speaking to me. Your Words are more precious to me than gold.

Jesus modeled a life of love and grace. He taught His disciples about developing a heart that loves God rather than robotically following rules. In Matthew 18:21, what does Peter ask Jesus about forgiveness?

The number seven is significant here; the Pharisees taught that after three times, you could stop forgiving someone. Peter doubled three and added one for good measure. Surely seven times was generous. But Jesus shocked him and the other disciples; how did He answer Peter's question in verse 22?

(The NIV translates this verse, "seventy-seven times;" it is translated "seventy times seven" in other translations.) Words in the Hebrew language have numerical value; tamin means the number 490 (7 X 70). Tamin refers to "complete," "perfect," or "finish."[2] If I stop forgiving, I am incomplete. The idea of keeping tallying of how many times I forgive people misses the point. Does God keep a record of my sins? How many times does He forgive me? Read Isaiah 43:25; what does God do with my sins?

Does God forget our sins? It's hard to imagine the omniscient Creator God forgetting something. This verse likely leans more toward the idea of not letting our sins affect our relationship with Him. Christ's blood covers our sin, and when we ask for forgiveness, God continually and unconditionally provides it.

Perhaps we can avoid a false refuge of bitterness if we develop a language of forgiveness. When we are offended, we don't have to stay there. We could respond, "God, empower me to forgive because You forgive me." When someone hurts us, we could respond, "God, that really hurt; give me courage to forgive, just as You forgive me when I hurt You." When the memory of the pain resurfaces, we could respond, "I thank You, Father, that you freed me from bitterness over that hurtful experience."

What remains unhealed will resurface. Refusing to forgive other people hurts you; forgiving heals you. Live in the freedom Jesus came to give us by forgiving those who hurt us just as He forgives us. Spend some time meditating on these words from Colossians 3:12-14: "Therefore, as God's chosen people, holy and dearly loved, clothe yourselves with compassion, kindness, humility, gentleness and patience. Bear with each other and forgive one another if any of you has a grievance against someone. Forgive as the Lord forgave you. And over all these virtues put on love, which binds them all together in perfect unity."

Record your response to your meditation on Colossians 3:12-14.

_____
_____
_____

Forgiveness is a holy practice that I need to embrace, Father. Keeping score is not Your way of loving me, and I want to love others in the same way. Help me choose forgiveness over bitterness and love over anger. I can only do that with Your help. Amen.

—— DAY 7: REFLECTION AND APPLICATION

Dear Lord, I delight in Your law and meditate on it day and night. Please plant me like a tree by streams of water, yielding fruit in season, keeping my leaves from withering, and prospering me in whatever I do for You.

As we have considered God's refuge of forgiveness, there have been many opportunities for reflection. Today put feet to your faith and take a practical step toward releasing any anger you have. It takes intention and persistence to embrace God as your refuge instead of choosing to remain angry.

Optional Journaling Prompts (choose one)
- Make a list of things that easily anger you. Pray God will help you process your anger in healthy ways. Ask Him to show you how to release your anger when it lingers too long. You might close your fists and imagine your anger in the palms of your hands. Then open your fists, saying, "I release my anger to You, Lord." Thank Him for taking your anger and replacing it with faith in Him and a peaceful spirit.
- Draw a horizontal line. On the left end of the line, write "Blame myself;" on the right side of the line, write "Blame others." Think about times when you blame yourself or others when a conflict arises. Put a dot on the line to represent where you think you fall on this spectrum most of the time. If you find you blame yourself more than others, put the dot more toward the left, or vice versa. Write about your participation in the "blame game," including why you think this practice has developed in your life. Pray for God's help in seeing the truth and releasing blame as a response to anger and fear.
- On Day 4 we looked at these steps for practicing true forgiveness. If you choose to use this procedure, record your thoughts and feelings about your experience.
    o Confront the offense
    o Confront the offender/offended
    o Release the revenge
- Make a two-column chart. Title the left side "Bitterness" and the right side "Grace." In each column create a list of what each of these look like for you and their results. Or locate images that represent each word and create two collages. Choosing grace is a way to break down the false refuge of bitterness and become better instead.
- You can develop a language of forgiveness by practicing, just as you learn any language. It may feel awkward at first, but it will become more natural the more you do it. Your language development may be internal only at first, but you may find ways to articulate your attitude of forgiveness in your speech and actions. These are examples you could use in your journal or create your own.
    o "I forgive _____ for _____ (hurt that was caused)."
    o "I choose to forgive _____, even though I don't yet feel like it."
    o "Thank You, God, for forgiving me. I forgive _____ for _____ just as you have forgiven me for _____."

- Read and record in your journal Genesis 50:20; in this verse, Joseph is putting the hurt his brothers caused him into a divine perspective. How has or can God use the pain of your life for good? What does a divine outlook of your trials look like? If you are not sure, ask God to show you and thank Him for helping you choose to become better rather than bitter by adopting His viewpoint.
- Find a song that encourages you in this process. You may document the lyrics and record your own reflections on them, or you could illustrate them with sketches or images you locate. Two examples for this week's theme song are "Better" by Jessica Reddy (2014) or "Lord, Make Me an Instrument of Thy Peace" by various artists, based on a prayer attributed to St. Francis of Assisi.

Remember to search for other's journal entries and post your own if you wish, using these hashtags on social media: #fp4h and #fp4hgodmyrefuge.

Precious Lord, thank You for Your refuge of unending love and mercy. Teach me to practice forgiveness in the same ways You freely offer it to me. I relinquish my perceived rights to my anger and desire for revenge, so that I can be filled with more of You. I humbly bow before You, my Creator and King. Amen.

Notes
1 Gregory Popcak, "Five Steps to Begin Overcoming Bitterness," March 28, 2019. https://brownpelicanla.com/five-steps-to-begin-overcoming-bitterness-by-dr-gregory-popcak/.
2 Jason Sobel, "Why 7 Times 70?" Fusion with Rabbi Jason, August 21, 2020. https://www.fusionglobal.org/connections/why-7-times-70/

Your Journaling

WEEK SEVEN: A REFUGE OF ACCEPTANCE

SCRIPTURE MEMORY VERSE
For you know the grace of our Lord Jesus Christ, that though he was rich, yet for your sake he became poor, so that you through his poverty might become rich. 2 Corinthians 8:9

Why do people overeat? There are many reasons for eating more than we need. Some people use eating to hide from painful emotions; food becomes a false refuge to avoid facing difficult emotions and memories. They might use it to avoid current unpleasant realities or to give themselves comfort. Overeating usually causes overweight. We live in a world where your appearance is evaluated to determine your worth. An overweight person can face ridicule, mocking, and shame. The person may respond by eating more and isolating. The cycle of eating and shame can be difficult to break.

You may be able to relate to this phenomenon. I lived this way myself. When I began to have weight problems after I turned six years old, I was teased and called names. I started to eat in an unconscious attempt to comfort myself, and the downward spiral began. My self-worth was wounded, and I began to believe that I would never be truly accepted unless I was thin instead of fat.

Last week we studied God's refuge of forgiveness; we looked at these truths.
- The desire for revenge and developing a bitter spirit will prevent us from healing from past pain.
- We can choose to allow anger to ferment or we can process and release it in healthy ways.
- Blaming ourselves or others perpetuates our anger and hurt and keeps us from healing.
- We can practice forgiveness by confronting the offense, confronting the offender or the offended, and releasing the desire for revenge.
- Practicing forgiveness is part of embracing God as our refuge and being free from bitterness.

This week we will examine how we view our bodies and how that lines up with how God sees us. We want to reject any shame and food addiction that traps us in cycles of despair and self-loathing. God created each of us as unique expressions of His image and His love. His refuge is one of full acceptance of His beloved children.

—— DAY 1: BODY SHAME

I'm thankful to meet with You today, Father. You have oceans of love to pour out on me, and I need Your help to face today's challenges. I open my heart to Your Word and Your Spirit.

How do we develop a negative view of our bodies? Our society plays a role. "In our contemporary culture, … we often automatically assume that a slender, delicately built woman with fine features is also a kind, smart, thoughtful and good person. We also believe that she is happy. Similarly, we consider that a physically strong, attractive man must be emotionally solid, dependable, upright and content."[1] These assumptions are lies; our character and worth are not related to exterior features.

When you look in the mirror at yourself, what grabs your attention?

_____
_____
_____

What does 1 Samuel 16:7 say about judging someone by outward appearance?

_____
_____

On Day 5 of Week 2's lesson, we looked at some scriptures that contain truths about our worth as God's creations. Review the chart of scripture verses and how each reflects your identity in Christ. What do you notice about these truths?

_____
_____

In order to leave a false refuge of shame, we must identify what caused us to enter it. Shame relates to our thoughts and feelings of worthlessness as a person, which is different from guilt we experience when we make a mistake or sin. What experiences have you had or do you presently have that cause you to feel shame?

_____
_____
_____

Let's see what God's Word says about shame and let His Spirit show us our true worth. Read each passage and record how it reveals your worth, using your name in place of the pronouns. The first one is done as an example.

Scripture	My Worth
Ephesians 2:4-7	God made Debbie alive when Debbie was dead, raised Debbie up with Christ, and seated Debbie in the heavenly realms in Him; He is showing Debbie the riches of His grace through Christ.
Isaiah 43:4a	
Luke 12:6-7	
Ephesians 1:4	
Ephesians 2:10	

Write a statement that expresses your worth to God based on these scriptures. Include your name in your statement.

_____
_____
_____
_____
_____

This process is one step in removing shame from our lives. This week we will continue to chip away at any shame and negative self-worth we may have. Be prayerful, asking God your refuge to make His truth known as you accept your true worth as His child

Thank You for the value You have placed in me as Your child. I rejoice that my worth is not based on my appearance or my performance but solely on what You say about me. Help me to recognize any shame or low self-worth that I have and replace them with Your view of me, a beloved child created to bear Your image in Your world. Amen.

DAY 2: YOUR BODY IMAGE

Make Your ways known to me, Lord; teach me Your paths. Guide me in Your truth and teach me, for You are the God of my salvation.

Some people are obsessed with how they look. Modern society provides a myriad of services to alter our appearances: plastic surgeons, hair colorists, Botox injections, nail spas, brow salons, and body sculptors. There's nothing wrong with taking care of yourself; a healthy level of self-care is good. But a hyper-focus on looks without satisfaction may stem from a negative self-image. "Body dysmorphia, or self-criticism for bodily imperfections that seem insignificant to someone else, is a common symptom of eating disorders. In its full blown form, body dysmorphic disorder (BDD) involves an obsessive *preoccupation with imagined or slight defects in appearance.*"[2] (emphasis added)

Yesterday we looked at our opinions of our bodies, whether positive or negative. Today we will honestly assess our bodies and see them through God's eyes. What part of your body do you think is your best feature? Why?

_____
_____
_____

What part of your body do you think is your least positive feature? Why?

_____
_____
_____

If you could change one thing about your body, what would it be?

_____
_____
_____

Read Psalm 139:13-16; what does verse 13 say about your body?

_____
_____
_____

How does the psalmist respond to this truth in verse 14?

_____
_____
_____

Do you believe that you are fearfully and wonderfully made? Sometimes I feel like my body is more fearful than wonderful! But my thoughts about myself, particularly about my body, reveal what I have learned, correctly or incorrectly, about my worth throughout my life. Being ridiculed about my weight as a child taught me that how much I weigh is the most important thing to consider when evaluating myself. It doesn't matter what other positive attributes I possess. I may try to compensate for my low self-worth by projecting a facade of confidence.

Instead of listening to the distortions of the world, the enemy, or my own inner thoughts, I need to see myself as God sees me. His Word is truth. Let's read what God says about our worth, since He is the One Who made us. As you read each passage, ask God to show you how valuable you are because you are His unique masterpiece.

Scripture	What God Says About My Uniqueness
Psalm 119:73-74	
Psalm 139:2-5	
Isaiah 64:8	
Romans 12:4-6	

What is unique about you that God is using or could use for His purposes?

_____
_____
_____

Fannie Crosby was a healthy newborn but at six months old, she was blinded by a quack doctor's treatment. Then her father died, and her mother had to work to support them. Fannie's godly grandmother was her caregiver. Although Fannie's eyes didn't allow her to see, God gifted her with an inner sight that allowed her to see Him in unique ways. She began writing poetry at age 8; here is her first poem.

> Oh, what a happy soul I am,
> although I cannot see!
> I am resolved that in this world
> Contented I will be.
>
> How many blessings I enjoy
> That other people don't,
> To weep and sigh because I'm blind
> I cannot, and I won't! [3]

During her lifetime, Fannie wrote the words to more than 9,000 hymns including "Blessed Assurance," "All the Way My Savior Leads Me," and "To God Be the Glory." Thankfully she was not focused on her lack of sight as her measure of self-worth. In fact, when a preacher said it was a shame God didn't give her sight along with her gift for writing, she responded, "Do you know that if at birth I had been able to make one petition, it would have been that I was born blind? Because when I get to heaven, the first face that shall ever gladden my sight will be that of my Savior."[4] She did not allow one part of her body to define her self-image; she saw herself through God's eyes.

If you believe you are worthless, you won't take care of yourself. Understanding your value as a person, as a creation of God, will help you see yourself as worthy of care, of love, and of purpose in the world. We will continue to work on that mental transformation tomorrow. For today let's thank God for creating us as unique and perfect in His sight.

Father, I reject the lie that my body is deficient and that my worth is measured by my appearance. I accept Your unique design for me, one of a kind, created for a specific purpose in Your plan. I am Yours, Father, and that is the best. Amen.

—— DAY 3: HEALTHY SELF-LOVE

Today is a day You have created, Lord, a day to worship You with my choices and praise You with my actions. Speak to me and lead me in Your wonderful ways

The Bible is full of direction about self-sacrifice and putting other's interests above our own. What does Philippians 2:3-4 say about this mindset?

_____
_____
_____

How do we balance following Christ's example of selflessness with a healthy love for ourselves? There is no command in the Bible to love yourself; it is assumed that we already do. Read Ephesians 5:29-30 and record what these verses say about self-love.

_____
_____
_____

Self-love is a given; in Mark 12:31 Jesus says to "love your neighbor as yourself." If you believe that your worth is sub-par, you are not believing the truth of God's view of you. God created you with purpose, love, and value. He desires fellowship with you and to be your refuge. I think that one reason we remain in a false refuge of pride is that we believe we are worthless and fear others will find out. Healthy self-love is seeing yourself as God sees you; self-love enhances love for Him and others.

1 Corinthians 13:4-7 is often read during wedding ceremonies. Let's take a fresh look at these verses; as you read them, record how you can love yourself. The first one is done as an example.

Verses	How I Can Love Myself
4	Patient: be kind to myself when I make the same mistake again and again, don't beat myself up. Just keep trying with God's help.
4	
4	

4	
4	
5	
5	
5	
5	
6	
7	
7	
7	
7	

Loving ourselves is part of loving God, because He loves us. We can learn to value what Christ values and seek to live by those values.

But how does loving ourselves relate to self-sacrifice and following Jesus? It is not the same as selfishness or self-indulgence. What does Jesus command His disciples to do in Matthew 16:24?

_____

_____

_____

Denying ourselves means putting our desires to the side and submitting to God's will. It doesn't mean thinking that we are insignificant. On the contrary, denying ourselves involves understanding our worth as we give ourselves to Him. A strong self-worth means you are giving God something you consider valuable. In Romans 12:1 we are told to be a "living sacrifice." Being a living sacrifice means you give the best to God, just as the Israelites gave the best of their flocks to God as a sacrifice. If I deny myself for His sake, it is of value because I am valuable. If I feel I'm worthless, what am I really giving Him?

Our memory verse talks about the greatest sacrifice ever made by the God Who loves you and considers you valuable enough to give His best. Use the blanks below to write out this week's memory verse, 2 Corinthians 8:9.

_____
_____
_____

Circle *grace*, *rich*, and *your sake*. If you trust Jesus for your salvation and follow Him, you are rich. If you feel that you are not worthy of love, you are missing the riches Christ has to offer you. Give yourself the same unconditional love God has for you and that He encourages us to have for others. Then you will focus on loving Him and others rather than yourself.

As we close this precious time with Him today, let's meditate on Psalm 34:5: "Those who look to Him are radiant with joy; their faces will never be ashamed."

Thank You, sweet Father, for making me in Your image to bear Your image to the world. I am greatly blessed and highly favored because I am Your child, lavished with love by Christ's sacrifice for me and filled with purpose to worship and witness about You. I love You so I can love myself and others. Amen.

—— DAY 4: REGRET INSTEAD OF REPROACH
Today I kneel before You, Righteous Judge and Holy God, because You are my King. You are God, and I am not, and as I spend time with You now, help me recognize that truth.

Last week we looked at the importance of forgiveness in embracing God's refuge. It is possible to forgive other people with God's help. But sometimes the person I need to forgive is myself. And that is an important part of loving myself. Remember that forgiveness is not earned; it is a gift. Look up Isaiah 1:18; how does God want to treat our sins?

_____
_____
_____

Confession is the start. Bring sin into the light so it can no longer have power over you. Once you have, it is finished. You may have consequences to live with, but God will be with you even in those situations. It is not necessary to bring up the sin again; it is covered by Christ's blood and you are forgiven. It is in the past, and *you can leave it there*. It doesn't define you; it is not your identity.

Read 2 Corinthians 5:21 and write it here.

_____
_____
_____

You have been transformed into the righteousness of God through Jesus. If you tend to berate yourself about things you did in the past, you can choose to say, "God has forgiven me, and I am forgiven." Our enemy loves to accuse us and keep us in bondage of self-imposed guilt. He doesn't want us to live in the freedom that forgiveness through Christ imparts.

Read Micah 7:19; what does this verse say about what God does with our sin?

_____
_____
_____

"When God buries our sins in the sea of forgetfulness, He then puts up a 'No Fishing' sign but many of us still insist on going back to try and bring them up again."[5] What does Psalm 103:11-12 say about God's treatment of our sin?

_____
_____
_____

Your sins are as far as the east is from the west. How far apart is that? On a globe, east and west never meet. If you replay past sins in your life and live in guilt and shame, you are on a never-ending journey that will drain you of energy and joy. Would you continue making a house payment once your mortgage was paid off? Isn't that the same as continuing to dwell on sins of the past that are forgiven through Christ? Your sin has been stamped "Forgiven;" the slate is wiped clean. Read Revelation 20:11-12. What is the scene and what happened to the people there?

_____
_____
_____

You may have encountered these verses before and shook in terror, thinking that your dark deeds are recorded in detail and will be made public at the end of time. The people in this scene are the lost, those who have rejected Jesus' gift of forgiveness. Read 2 Timothy 4:8 and Revelation 3:5; what is different about the Christian's experience?

_____
_____

If we are saved through Jesus, we will be rewarded for what we have done for Christ since our salvation. We will not be judged for our sin. Your name is written in God's Book of Life, and nothing can erase your name from that ledger. That's the only record that matters. He is intent on loving you and walking with you daily as you live in liberty. "Forgiveness is the principal activity and heart attitude needed to pave the way for freedom."[6]

We can choose to exchange reproach with regret. Regret means to feel a sense of loss; it doesn't involve condemnation or reliving the pain of past failures. As I look at my past, I don't say, "I was so stupid; I'll never do any better. I hate myself." Instead I say, "I regret that I made that choice. But God has forgiven me, and I forgive myself." We can grieve over the mistakes, and we can leave them behind. We can face them honestly, forgive ourselves, and move forward.

In *Enter Wild*, Carlos Whittaker talks about forgiving all parts of yourself, even the parts that sin and make your life harder. You may need to apologize to the parts of yourself you have hated and condemned.[7] What parts of your body or your being need your forgiveness?

_____
_____
_____

My dear Father, I can be hard on myself. I expect perfection and constantly disappoint myself. I have sins in my past that cause me grief. I trust that Christ has done the work for me on the cross, and as I confess my sins, You forgive them. Help me replace reproach with regret. Amen.

—— DAY 5: DELIVERANCE

Today I enter into Your presence with anticipation, Lord. I find my strength and my purpose in You alone. Speak to my heart and teach me Your truths.

Perhaps your struggle with making healthy choices comes from a struggle with loving yourself, living in a false refuge to protect your self-worth since you think you are not valuable. You may believe that you are not worthy of love because of something you have done in the past. Today we will confront the lies and replace them with the truth of how much God loves and values you.

Let's read the story of a woman who faced public shame and condemnation. As we do, see the story from her viewpoint. Read John 8:2-3. What situation does the woman find herself in?

_____
_____
_____

Stand in her place; she cowered before Jesus, guilty of breaking one of the Ten Commandments. How would you feel? Ashamed? Afraid? In verses 4-6 what do we learn about the Jewish leaders' reason for bringing her to Jesus?

_____
_____
_____

Once again put yourself in her place; how would you feel to learn you are being used as a pawn in a power struggle? Her dignity and worth have been stripped from her, and she likely feels cheap and expendable. But then Jesus spoke and changed everything. What did He tell the Jewish leaders (verse 7)?

_____
_____
_____

Jesus knew their intent. He got to the heart of the matter; *we all sin*. They were no different from her and had no right to judge her. He took her guilt and applied it to them as well. She saw that Jesus didn't consider her less than the powerful self-righteous men. After they all left, Jesus asked her a question. What is the question, and how does she respond (verses 10-11)?

_____
_____
_____

Her accusers were gone; Jesus can do the same for us. He can take the accusers out of our minds and deliver us from the constant barrage of lies that seek to condemn us. He can restore our self-worth and dignity, because when He looks at us, He sees us through eyes of love and mercy. What were Jesus' final words to her in verse 11?

_____
_____
_____

Jesus told her that she could choose to see herself through His eyes and leave the past behind. He didn't define her by her adultery, whether it was a one-time act or a lifestyle. What does that look like for me? I can choose to identify myself as Debbie the divorcée, Debbie the fatty, Debbie the too-shy-to-speak-up-for-herself, or whatever my current mistake or crisis wants to call me. Or I can embrace my imperfections; recognize them, don't deny them. I can develop a value system that understands my worth based on God's love. Read Psalm 8:3-4. What does the psalmist say about humanity in light of God's majesty?

_____
_____
_____

Yet where has God put us in the hierarchy of creation (verses 5-8)?

_____
_____
_____

He has made us co-rulers of His creation. You are royalty, not because of what you have done or what others think about you, but because of God's design. If He could love me as a rebellious sinner, caught in the act of sin on a regular basis, He can help me learn to love myself. I want to be delivered from the lie that says I'm not good enough and abide in His refuge of acceptance.

Going through a separation and divorce forced me to face the fact that I didn't love myself. I depended on others to affirm me, and I based my worth on accomplishments. When the person I loved most rejected me and I faced the failure of my marriage, those two sources of my validation disappeared. God taught me to love myself despite my rejection and failure. About six years after my divorce was final, I was walking at the mall and suddenly felt a release within me, like a weight was lifted from my shoulders. I don't know another way to describe it. But I knew what it meant. After a lot of work and prayer, I finally accepted myself the way I was: my failures, sin, recovering overeater, perfectionist, shy, and wounded. I knew who I was and loved myself as God does. I left my false refuge of self-loathing and shame, and I found acceptance in His perfect refuge. Praise God for going with me through that valley and bringing me out on the other side, healed and whole. I am convinced in the core of my being that my value is based solely on what God says about me, not the opinion of others or my achievements. You can know that, too. How are you learning or have learned to accept yourself as God does?

_____

_____

_____

Thank You, Lord, for restoring my value and dignity. I want to be delivered from the attacks against my identity as Your beloved created child. Help me participate with You in the process of fully abiding in You my refuge. I praise You for Your power and Your holiness. Amen.

—— DAY 6: REFLECTION AND APPLICATION
Holy Lord, my mind is swirling with thoughts and distractions. Remove everything that keeps me from focusing on You right now. I want to hear You and know You more.

Exploring one's self-worth can be painful and confusing. If you struggle with low self-esteem, let God open your heart to His healing love and believe the value He places on you. You are a child of the King and the apple of His eye, and His truth about your significance can set you free.

As you develop healthier self-love, you begin to accept yourself more easily. Ironically the more accepting you are of yourself, the strength of the false refuge of pride fades. You are more available to authentically love others and be used in mighty ways by God. Loving yourself is a blessing, allowing you to become all God created you to be. You may experience rejection, but that does not mean you are rejected as a person. You can choose to see the rejection separate from your self-worth. Jesus was rejected by religious experts. Those who knew God's Word the best hated Him the most. They were responsible for killing Him. What does Isaiah 53:3 say about the way Jesus was treated while here on earth?

Read Matthew 27:46; what was Jesus' cry to His Father?

Jesus' rejection resulted in our acceptance. Practice this week's memory verse here.

Reflect on your worth in Christ and your love for yourself. What have you learned this week that will have the greatest impact on your ability to love yourself?

What do you still need to accept and love yourself the way God your refuge does?

I want to end today's lesson by giving you a big virtual hug. I'm praying God is wrapping His arms around you right now, and that you know He is with you, loves you, and is holding you close. His love for you will never fail, and I pray your love for yourself mirrors His unconditional love for you.

Thank You for holding me in Your arms, Lord. I'm very glad You have chosen to accept me based on Jesus' sacrifice for me; help me to accept myself as You do. I want to love You and others more, and I know Your love for me will never fail. I am overwhelmingly blessed to be Your child. Amen.

DAY 7: REFLECTION AND APPLICATION
My life is in Your hands, Father. I yield my will to Yours and bow before You now, knowing that this time with You is the best part of my day. I'm ready to hear You speak to me.

This week we have focused on God's refuge of acceptance. During your reflection time today, choose an activity that suits you best as you have encountered truths about your worth and your beliefs about yourself.

Optional Journaling Prompts (choose one)
- Locate a recent photo of yourself. Honestly assess your appearance, putting aside what others say about you. Starting at the top of your head and moving down to your toes, thank God specifically for each part of your body. Then write down all the things you like about yourself.
- Create a two-column chart. On one side write down what the world says is beautiful, and on the other side write down what God says is beautiful. Include specific scriptures if you like.
- Write a love letter to yourself. Tell yourself how you are the apple of God's eye and how much He loves you. Use wording from the scriptures we've studied this week.
- Create a list of mistakes or sins in your life that still haunt you. Write over the list diagonally in bold letters, "Paid in Full." Thank God for removing your sin and covering it with Jesus' blood. Ask for His help to let go of any guilt and shame and replace it with regret.
- Find a song that encourages you in this process. You may document the lyrics and record your own reflections on them, or you could illustrate them with sketches or images you locate. Two examples for this week's theme song are "You Say" by Lauren Daigle (2018) or "Fingerprints of God" by Steven Curtis Chapman (2013).

Remember to search for other's journals and post your own if you wish, using these hashtags on social media: #fp4h and #fp4hgodmyrefuge.

Sweet Father, thank You for creating me as Your unique child, a reflection of Your image, and deeply loved just as I am. Help me to continue to develop my self-love as You work in me to reveal Christ's image; thank You for Your refuge of acceptance where I can abide. I love You. Amen.

Your Journaling

Notes

1 F. Diane Barth, "What's the Best Way to Deal With a Negative Body Image?" Psychology Today: July 7, 2015. https://www.psychologytoday.com/us/blog/the-couch/201507/whats-the-best-way-deal-negative-body-image.

2 Ibid.

3 Mark Galli (ed.), "Fanny Crosby: Prolific and Blind Hymn Writer," October 1, 2020. https://www.christianitytoday.com/history/people/poets/fanny-crosby.html.

4 Ibid.

5 Jack Wellman, "How To Forgive Yourself: A Christian Commentary." https://www.whatchristianswanttoknow.com/how-to-forgive-yourself-a-christian-commentary/.

6 Chester Kylstra, Biblical Healing and Deliverance: A Guide to Experiencing Freedom from Sins of the Past, Destructive Beliefs, Emotional and Spiritual Pain, Curses and Oppression (Ada, MI: Chosen Books, 2014) 33.

7 Carlos Whittaker, op. cit, 129.

WEEK EIGHT: A REFUGE OF JOY

SCRIPTURE MEMORY VERSE
For you shall go out in joy and be led forth in peace; the mountains and the hills before you shall break forth into singing, and all the trees of the field shall clap their hands. Isaiah 55:12

I live in southeast Texas on the Gulf Coast. If you are not familiar with that area, I can give you a word to describe it: flat. As far as the eye can see, there is almost no change in the elevation of the landscape. Imagine my experience when I visited Colorado Springs. Every morning I woke up and saw enormous mountains framing the window. Wherever we drove, there were mountains around every corner. We drove to the top of Pikes Peak (Don't do it; take the cog railway instead!), and I stood at the very top of the mountain, filled with jaw-dropping awe at the majestic view.

We have all had mountaintop experiences in our faith journey. We've had times when we felt very close to God and times we had a revelation about our relationship with Him. We have found joy and communion with Him beyond the norm. Those times are precious and exciting, and they can be times God uses to speak to us and prepare us for what is coming next. We love being on the mountains with Him, sitting in His presence and soaking up His majesty. This is a part of God's refuge, and it a refuge of joy.

Last week we studied God's refuge of acceptance and explored these ideas.
- We may experience shame because of our self-image, but God sees us as His good creation.
- Each person is unique with special gifts and attributes from God that make us precious in His sight.
- There is a healthy balance between self-sacrifice and self-love/care.
- We can choose regret over our past failures instead of self-reproach.
- Jesus offers deliverance from self-condemnation and restores our dignity and worth.

Our study this week will focus on experiencing joy in God. Once we have left a false refuge behind, we experience a mountaintop high. How can we continue experiencing joy in God our refuge after the excitement of mountaintop experiences wanes?

—— DAY 1: JOURNEY TO THE MOUNTAINTOP

My Father, how I love to spend quiet time alone with You. I want to hear Your voice, to know You more, to experience Your presence in a new way. Thank You for meeting with me now; I'm ready to listen.

Rock climbers enjoy the process of scaling a wall and reaching the summit. They experience a view that is preceded by specific training that prepares them for the climb. In our spiritual walk, we sometimes have mountains to climb. Our goals to lose weight and achieve fitness may be one of those mountains. And the process may be difficult for us to embrace. But we may choose to embrace the climb as we work toward our goals.

The prophet Elijah learned about scaling mountains. Read 1 Kings 17:1. When Elijah bursts on the scene in the Northern Kingdom of Israel, what does he announce to King Ahab?

_____
_____
_____

After he leaves the king's presence, where does God send him? (verses 2-3)

_____
_____
_____

How did God provide for him? (verses 4-6)

_____
_____
_____

God was training Elijah for a future mountain-top experience. Elijah's first lesson was to obey God and *walk in faith*. He didn't question God when He told him to confront evil king Ahab with terrible news, a task that could have resulted in his death. He didn't question God when He told him to go and hide himself in the Kerith Ravine on the farthest western border of Israel's land. The name for this location means a separation or cutting; God was truly separating Elijah from his comfort zone! He accepted the food and drink God had provided through unusual circumstances. May we have that kind of faith with our daily food plan and intake, trusting God that He will provide and that the First Place for Health food plan helps us reach our goals. May we separate ourselves from the world and its call to take shortcuts to lose weight, only to return to unhealthy habits.

What happened to our mountain-climber next? Read 1 Kings 17:7; after some time, Elijah faced what situation?

Read verse 8; where did God send Elijah next?

How did God provide food for Elijah and for the woman who took him in? (verses 10-16)

The second thing Elijah learned was to *depend on God for everything*. Although he was God's prophet and obeying Him, he had to live through drought conditions with everyone else. Yet God provided for him in miraculous and unexpected ways during those tough times. He sent Elijah to a town away from his own country, further west than the Kerith Ravine. The name of the town Zarephath comes from a word that means a place for smelting metal. As we prepare to scale mountains, God our refuge can use every experience to make us stronger and more dependent on Him. He may use our struggles with making healthy choices to form us into the people He created us to become.

Over three years passed, and the time came for the drought to end. Elijah returned to confront the king and those who followed the pagan god Baal. He met first with Obadiah, one of the prophets of God, and told him to go and get King Ahab. What did Obadiah say to Elijah in 1 Kings 18:9-14?

The third thing we can learn from Elijah's training is to *expect opposition from others*. Even someone who follows God can misunderstand the path God has called you to take. Don't be surprised when some don't support your unique journey. Keep your focus on God and don't let them discourage you or move you from the way God is leading you.

Elijah called the king and pagan prophets to meet him on a mountain, Mount Carmel. Turn to 1 Kings 18 to read about this amazing "Battle of the Gods." What challenge did Elijah throw down to Baal's prophets in verses 22-24?

_____
_____
_____

In verses 25-29 the prophets of Baal had their turn with their sacrifice. What happened in their part of the challenge?

_____
_____
_____

In verses 30-35 Elijah had his turn and prepared the sacrifice for the Lord God. He poured enormous amounts of water over the altar, although they lived through a three-and-a-half year drought! The water was likely undrinkable, but the irony is there.

What happened to the sacrifice that Elijah presented to God? (verses 36-38)

_____
_____
_____

What was the response of the people in verse 39?

_____
_____
_____

Finally, we learn from Elijah that the *mountaintop experience is to honor God*. It is all about Him and bringing other people to Him. He wants everyone to know Him and have a relationship with Him (2 Peter 3:9). We may become self-absorbed and forget that our mountaintop journey and experience is about Him and not us. As you follow all the parts of this program and lose weight, you will have amazing opportunities to share what God has done in your life. Be careful to give Him praise and use those occasions to witness about His power and love.

Our lessons from Elijah are:
- obey God and walk in faith;
- depend on God for everything;
- expect opposition from others; and
- remember the mountaintop experience is to honor God.

On each step of Elijah's journey toward Mount Carmel, he chose to hope in God and trust Him for the outcome, even though he didn't know the specific events that he would face. Leaving the outcome in the hands of God, moving forward as He leads, step by step, day by day, and trusting Him consistently results in dwelling in His refuge of joy.

Which one of these four lessons is most meaningful to you at this point on your wellness journey? Why?

_____
_____
_____

Thank You, Lord, for being with me every step of the way up the mountains in my life. Help me use these lessons from Elijah's journey as I learn to love You more and trust You completely with my mind, spirit, emotions, and body. Amen.

—— DAY 2: TIME OF REFRESHMENT

My time with You, Father, is precious. My life is full of distractions and busyness that moves my focus away from You. Give me a clear mind and undivided heart as I sit in Your presence now; speak to me as only You can.

Mountaintop experiences often come after a struggle in life. Elijah had struggled for three and a half years to stay in hiding from angry King Ahab and survive a drought. God provided for him and the woman and child with whom he lived, but there were drought conditions all the same. However, now he was on the mountaintop, and God defeated his enemies.

Read 1 Kings 18:41-43. What did Elijah tell King Ahab in verse 41?

_____
_____

What did Elijah do in verse 42?

___

What command did Elijah give his servant in verse 43?

___

What happened in verses 44-45?

___

What did Elijah do in verse 46?

___

Several things in these verses show us truths about mountaintop experiences. First, Elijah knew that God would bring the rain. He bowed his face to the ground, humbling himself before God. He understood that even on the mountaintop, God is God and he is His servant. Next, he waited patiently for God's perfect timing. Why did God make him wait? Perhaps God was developing patience in his servant. Certainly, God could have sent the rain at any time. But He didn't do it immediately. God is sovereign, knowing the right time for everything. Finally, Elijah received amazing power from God. He outran the king's chariot back to the city, about 17 miles! Remember that Elijah had lived through drought conditions before this encounter on Mount Carmel, so this power came directly from God. That is strength I could use!

Elijah did the following on the mountaintop.
- Humbled himself before God (He "bent down to the ground and put his face between his knees.")
- Waited on God (He sent his servant back to look at the sea seven times before a cloud was visible.)
- Received enormous power from God. ("The power of the Lord came on Elijah and... he ran... all the way to Jezreel.")

As we continue on our wellness journey, we will have times of refreshing mountaintop experiences. There will be times when we faithfully follow all the aspects of this program, and we will see God blessing us with progress. Continue to bow before God your refuge, wait for His timing, and draw all your strength from Him. Those are characteristics of a mountaintop dweller!

How is God developing these characteristics in you? How are they helping you, or how could they help you, in your wellness journey?

Humility _____

Patience _____

Strength _____

Father, thank You for showering me with all that I need. Give me humility to bow before You, patience to wait for Your timing, and strength to do all You want me to do. I love You and trust You. Amen.

—— DAY 3: PERILS OF PRIDE

My heart is longing today, Father. I have needs and desires that only You can fill. Help me to open my ears and my eyes to all that You want to say and show to me.

After Elijah's experience, defeating the prophets of Baal and seeing God bring rain after three and a half years of drought, you might think that he would literally be on cloud nine! But mountaintop experiences do not ensure a permanent feeling of euphoria. In fact, we have to be very careful that we do not fall prey to the false refuge that has been on our radar since the beginning of this study – pride.

Read 1 Kings 19:1-4. Why did Elijah run for his life?

_____

_____

_____

Elijah escaped and went on a one day journey into the wilderness (verse 4). What did he tell God? _

_____

_____

_____

How did God respond to Elijah's words in verses 5-7?

Then what was Elijah able to do (verse 8-9)?

Notice that Elijah ran away from danger after he arrived back in Jezreel. But this time he didn't run in the strength of the Lord. He ran in his own strength. And he went to the wilderness, which is often used in scripture as a metaphor for a time of testing (e.g., Israel's wandering it the wilderness for forty years and Jesus' temptation in the wilderness). We have to be careful that we are not so excited by our mountaintop experience that we begin to operate in our own power. As we progress on our wellness journey, it is easy to forget that it is God Who is accomplishing His work in us. When you receive compliments on your weight loss, be careful not to puff up with pride but to humbly thank God and give Him the glory.

God gave Elijah food that strengthened him enough to travel for forty days. I wish that was something available in my grocery store! When God nourishes us – body, soul, mind, and spirit – we have everything we need to accomplish His work in and through us. The food plan we are using is enough to fill us and give us the strength we need to live every day. We may think we need more food and get hungry at times. But we can trust God to use the food He provides to fuel us completely.

If you struggle with hunger pains, you might try this strategy that has helped me. As I prepare to eat a meal or snack, I hold my open hand, palm down over the food. I pray to God, thanking Him for this specific food that He has provided, and that this food will sustain me, satisfy my hunger, and will be enough for me until I eat again. If I feel or think I am hungry before my next meal, I recall that prayer and thank Him that He is enough for all my hunger pangs and all my needs.

Elijah encountered another peril of pride from his mountaintop experience. Read 1 Kings 19 verses 10 and 14. What does he say to God?

Maybe you feel like you are the Lone Ranger. When you go out to eat with friends, you are the only one making healthy choices. While others are sleeping in, you are out hitting the pavement exercising. And it is easy to whine and complain: "God, why did you make me this way? Why do I have to work incredibly hard at losing weight when others don't have to do it?"

That is pride talking! Elijah forgot that God was the One Who caused the drought, the One Who provided for him during the drought, and the One Who gave him a part in defeating the prophets of Baal. God was the One Who brought the rain and empowered Elijah to run faster than a horse-drawn chariot for 17 miles. Things didn't go the way Elijah expected after that, so he ran away to hide and have a pity party. Can we relate?

How did God respond to Elijah's complaints in 1 Kings 19:18?

___

Dear friend, isn't it wonderful to know that we are not alone on our wellness journey? In First Place for Health, we travel with other fitness seekers, and we support each other along the way. At a recent meeting our members were sharing prayer requests and drawing names for our weekly prayer partners. I contacted someone who was absent first thing the next morning to tell her who her prayer partner would be for that week. She said the person who had drawn her name had already contacted her! That is the kind of fellowship and loyal support this program can offer us. But you can't isolate yourself in the wilderness as Elijah did; you must stay in close contact with your team members and leader. We need each other; there is no room for pride.

How has pride been a challenge for you on your wellness journey?

___

How does having a First Place for Health group support you, and how do you support your group? Give some specific examples you have experienced.

___

Father, I know that you despise pride, and I do not want my pride to keep me from following You. Give me a humble heart and let me know when I'm falling into a prideful mindset. You are everything to me, and I trust You to be in control of my life. Amen.

—— DAY 4: EXPERIENCING GOD
It's good to draw away from my to-do list and put all my focus on You, Lord. Take this time we have together and make it all You want it to be for Your glory and my good.

Elijah went from drought to victory on Mount Carmel, to the wilderness and to another mountain. In 1 Kings 19:8-9, where was Elijah?

Here Mount Horeb is called "the mountain of God." This place is historic for several reasons.
- Moses met God here and saw the burning bush. (Exodus 3)
- Many scholars believe that Horeb was another name for Sinai, which is the mountain where Moses met God and received the Ten Commandments and the law for His people, the Israelites (Exodus 19-24). It's possible that it was one mountain but had different names for opposite sides.
- Horeb is thought to mean "glowing heat."

On Mount Horeb, Elijah has a new encounter with God. Read 1 Kings 19:11-13; what does God tell Elijah to do (verse 11)?

In verses 11-12, Elijah experiences four things as he waits for God to "pass by." What are the four ways God revealed Himself to Elijah in these verses?
1.
2.
3.
4.

How did Elijah respond (verse 13)?

Elijah came from a wilderness of depression, fear, and loneliness to a second mountaintop. God ministered to him by feeding him, giving him rest, and calling him to meet Him at Mount Horeb. Elijah obeyed God, even though he was feeling down. Perhaps you've felt that way on your wellness journey. You may have worked hard and followed the program but didn't see much or any weight loss for a long time. It's easy to get discouraged on this path of following God our refuge and trusting Him for the results. But He continually offers a refuge of joy despite the difficult circumstances.

Elijah found God in a quiet place. God knew how to speak to him at this moment, in this place. God spoke to people in many ways throughout the Bible. He spoke to Job from a storm (Job 38), Moses from a burning bush (Exodus 3), and Paul from a light from heaven (Acts 9). Those are dramatic revelations and what we often consider "mountaintop" experiences. But sometimes God speaks in a whisper. On Mount Horeb between the wilderness and Elijah's next assignment, God pulled him aside to whisper to him. What was the purpose of the wind, earthquake, and fire? Maybe God wanted Elijah to see that the drama of Mount Carmel wasn't the only way he could hear God's voice. The loud noises and movement of the first three events surely was startling in contrast to the deafening silence of God speaking in a whisper in complete stillness.

We may experience God on a mountaintop, but it won't always be a big, dramatic show with a crowd of people, a soundtrack, and fireworks. When He speaks to us in the quiet stillness of our hearts, it is just as real, meaningful, and valid as those outwardly sensational events. We can have small mountaintop experiences every day as we come alone into God's presence, faces covered as we encounter the glowing light of His glory, expecting to find Him in even the smallest, quietest whispers of the Spirit in our hearts. He will speak to us within His refuge of joy, found only in His presence.

How has God spoken to you in the past that was big and dramatic? Record a specific experience.

How has God spoken to you in quiet ways? Record a specific experience.

Where are you today in your wellness journey in relationship to a mountaintop experience with God? What is He calling you to do in order to meet Him and listen to His voice?

Thank You, holy Father, for speaking to me in whispers meant just for me through Your Spirit in my soul. I need to hear Your voice and know You more. May I experience You in a new, fresh way as I seek You first. Amen.

—— DAY 5: PREPARING FOR NEW CHALLENGES
Thank You for this day, dear Lord, and for time to spend with You. As I am in Your presence right now, still my busy mind and open my needy heart to hear Your voice and know Your love.

Elijah went through two dramatic mountaintop experiences. He battled and defeated the prophets of Baal with crowds of people and lightning from heaven. He experienced God all alone in the wind, an earthquake, fire, and a whisper. Both mountaintop experiences were memorable, meaningful, and involved a message.

Open to 1 Kings 19:15-17. What did God tell Elijah in this passage?

God's message to Elijah started with, "Go back the way you came." God had more challenges ahead for Elijah and his ministry. And he couldn't do those things on the mountaintop. It is hard to leave a mountaintop experience with God; we want to stay and continue communing with Him. But we must return to the real world. The same challenges will be there as well as new challenges. But we have been strengthened and empowered by our time with God, and He equips us to not only face the challenges but to be victorious.

Consider the mountaintop experiences you've had in the past. How did God use them to equip you for the next part of your faith journey?

There is a thread that runs throughout the Old Testament. It starts with Moses and Joshua. Imagine what it would be like to take Moses' place as the leader of the Israelites. Moses had been God's hand in the ten plagues of Egypt, the parting of the Red Sea, bringing water from a rock, establishing the law and building the tabernacle, and leading the people for over forty years. Joshua had big shoes to fill! He may have felt inadequate. But God trained him for years and continually gave Joshua encouragement.

Read Deuteronomy 31:6-7 and verse 23. What phrase does Moses repeat in these verses?

Why could the people "be strong and courageous?"

Let's look at some other examples of this phrase of support. In the following passages you will find the phrase, "Be strong and courageous." Who was encouraging whom and why?

Scripture	Who Encouraged Whom	Why
Joshua 1:1, 6-9, 18		
Joshua 10:5, 25		

Scripture	Who Encouraged Whom	Why
2 Samuel 2:4-7		
1 Chronicles 19:10-13		
1 Chronicles 22:11-13 1 Chronicles 28:20		
2 Chronicles 32:1, 7-8		

God's people internalized this encouraging phrase from God and used it over and over again throughout their history. He wanted them to remember that He was their refuge, was always with them, and would give them victory over their enemies when they were obedient to Him. How does this phrase, "Be strong and courageous," impact you? How can God use this encouragement in your life?

Jesus continually encouraged His disciples with the phrases, "Don't be afraid" and "Fear not." It is one of the most common commands in the Bible. That might mean that we tend to be afraid and need that reminder, that God is always with us, and that we can trust Him, hope in Him, and find joy in Him.

After you leave the mountaintop, He doesn't stay on the mountaintop while you climb down alone. He goes with you. He never leaves you. As you develop a healthy lifestyle, lean on Him every moment. Take the joy from the mountaintop with you and let it be your constant companion. No matter what challenges lie ahead, God your refuge has been there before you, prepared the way, and will take every step with you. "Be strong and courageous!"

Close out your time with God today by practicing your memory verse.

"Be strong and take heart, all you who hope in the Lord." Psalm 31:24

God, I'm thankful that You are always with me, giving me strength and courage to face every challenge in my life. Help me as I lean on You for all I need and find wonderful joy in the Name of God, the Great I Am. Amen.

—— DAY 6: REFLECTION AND APPLICATION
Thank You, Father, for the opportunity to be in Your presence right now. I eagerly anticipate hearing what Your Word has to say to me and experiencing Your loving arms around me as I spend time with You.

Not long after the birth of our second child, my husband told me that he wanted to transfer from Houston to Dallas. I was caring for a newborn and an almost four-year-old. I would leave my support system: family, friends, and my church home who were dear to me. I would leave my First Place group. His news came out of the blue. But the moment he told me about these plans, I immediately had peace. God assured me that I didn't have to be afraid of these changes, and I could be strong and take courage. I never doubted that God my refuge was in control and would provide. A few months later my husband and I separated. Even then I knew God was supporting and caring for us. I lived in His refuge of joy as I dwelt in His presence.

How has God provided a refuge of joy for you when you faced uncertain circumstances?
_____
_____
_____

How has God's Word been a source of strength and comfort during these times?
_____
_____
_____

List three verses or passages that are meaningful to you as you reflect on these experiences.
1. _____
2. _____
3. _____

Isaiah 55:11 says, "So is my word that goes out from my mouth: It will not return to me empty, but will accomplish what I desire and achieve the purpose for which I sent it." How has God accomplished His purposes in you through His Word? __

God's presence is the refuge of joy that provides hope in the face of adversity and peace in the midst of trials. We can experience God every day because of His grace and mercy, through the Holy Spirit within us. Let us thank Him for His indescribable gift and seek Him first in everything!

I'm deeply grateful for Your Word, dear Lord, and how You use it to accomplish Your purposes in me and in the world. I know Your Word will never fail and that I can depend on its truth. Amen.

—— DAY 7: REFLECTION AND APPLICATION

Holy Father, You are my all in all. I need You every minute of every day. As I come before You now, fill me with Your Spirit and work in my heart to put me more in line with Your purposes.

When Ezekiel was on the mountain with God, he saw His glory. No one can experience the presence and glory of God and remain the same. As you reflect on this week's study, consider how your experiences with God have changed you. How has He made you more Christ-like? You have many mountains yet to climb, and He is with you on every step of your journey. He offers His refuge of joy all along the way. Reflect on this refuge of joy and how experiencing God is changing you.

Optional Journaling Prompts (choose one)
- Locate images of mountains and views from tops of mountains in print or online. Paste them in your journal and write captions for each that represent how you feel in God's presence during a mountaintop experience.
- Think about mountaintop experiences you have had in the past. Reflect on how you got to the mountaintop. Draw a line that shows an upward movement, and write down the events that took place on your way to the mountaintop.
- Find a song that encourages you in this process. You may document the lyrics and record your own reflections on them, or you could illustrate them with sketches or images you locate. Two examples are "Show Me Your Glory" by Third Day (2001) and "The God on the Mountain" by Tracy Dartt (1975).

O Lord, I desire to be with You on the mountaintop, Your refuge of joy, to draw away from the world, see Your face, and hear Your voice. May I be open to Your movement in my life as You draw me near to You. Renew and strengthen me to serve You with my whole heart. Amen.

Your Journaling

WEEK NINE: A TIME TO CELEBRATE

During this study we have examined many ways that God provides refuge. We've learned about false refuges, why we might flee to them, and how we can exchange them for God's true refuge. Our goal has been to strengthen our dependence on Him and know Him more. This week you will reflect on how God has spoken to you during this session. To help you shape your short victory celebration testimony, work through the following questions in your prayer journal, one on each day leading up to your group's celebration.

DAY ONE: List some of the benefits you have gained by allowing the Lord to transform your life through this twelve-week First Place for Health session. Be mindful that He has been active in all four aspects of your being, so list benefits you have received in the physical, mental, emotional and spiritual realms.

DAY TWO: In what ways have you most significantly changed mentally? Have you seen a shift in the ways you think about yourself, food, your relationships, or God? How has Scripture memory been a part of these shifts?

DAY THREE: In what ways have you most significantly changed emotionally? Have you begun to identify how your feelings influence your relationship to food and exercise? What are you doing to stay aware of your emotions, both positive and negative?

DAY FOUR: In what ways have you most significantly changed spiritually? How has your relationship with God deepened? How has drawing closer to Him made a difference in the other three areas of your life?

DAY FIVE: In what ways have you most significantly changed physically? Have you met or exceeded your weight/measurement goals? How has your health improved during the past twelve weeks?

DAY SIX: Was there one person in your First Place for Health group who was particularly encouraging to you? How did their kindness make a difference in your First Place for Health journey?

DAY SEVEN: Summarize the previous six questions into a one-page testimony, or "faith story," to share at your group's victory celebration.

May our Mighty God make you victorious in Him, as you continue to keep Him first in all things!

LEADER DISCUSSION GUIDE

For in-depth information, guidance and helpful tips about leading a successful First Place for Health group, spend time studying the *My Place for Leadership* book. In it, you will find valuable answers to most of your questions, as well as personal insights from many First Place for Health group leaders.

For the group meetings in this session, be sure to read and consider each week's discussion topics several days before the meeting—some questions and activities require supplies and/or planning to complete. Also, if you are leading a large group, plan to break into smaller groups for discussion and then come together as a large group to share your answers and responses. Make sure to appoint a capable leader for each small group so that discussions stay focused and on track (and be sure each group records their answers!).

—— WEEK ONE: A REFUGE OF ABUNDANCE

Locate an image of a stronghold from David's time (1003-970 BC). Discuss how this structure could provide refuge for someone fleeing from an enemy. How does God provide refuge for us in a similar way?

Ask members to share times of scarcity, real or perceived, they have experienced. How did God show up? What did He do to reveal His abundance?

How do we use God's Word to access His power? What does your daily interaction with God's Word and His presence look like? How does His Word impact and change you?

Ask a member to read Colossians 3:1-3. An abundant life-liver "sets [her] mind on things above, not on things below." What are the "things above" and how do you keep your mind focused them? Paul's life is an example of an abundant life, but it was not a bed of roses. What are positive aspects about living an abundant life in Christ? What are the challenging aspects?

Encourage members to share experiences where they fully trusted God and how He honored their faith. How can we avoid King Jeroboam's lack of faith and gain total rather than partial victory, especially in our fitness journey?

Ask members to share how they used the Day 6 and 7 reflections to deepen their understanding about God's refuge and applying that understanding in their lives.

Close by reading the Day 7 prayer over your group. Or lead the group members in a choral reading; they can insert their names where appropriate.

—— WEEK TWO: REFUGE OF TRUTH

Read Helen Baratta's story from the beginning of this week's study. Ask members to share any personal connections they have to her story. Read the excerpt from Day 7 and ask members to share their stories of deliverance.

Ask a member to read Psalm 62:5-8 aloud. How do David's words reflect God's refuge in members' lives? Where do members want to find refuge in God?

Forgiveness and unforgiveness are two sides to the same coin. Ask members to describe the importance of forgiveness in their own lives and how that is part of their spiritual practices. Ask members to share how they deal with forgiving others and any barriers they have to overcome to forgive difficult people in their lives.

Ask members to share any lies they uncovered during this week's study. How has God's Word helped them identify and confront these lies? How has members' families impacted their lives in ways that have either created or prevented a false refuge to form?

Our identity in Christ is a foundation for building a life that abides in God as the true refuge. Refer to the chart of verses in the Day 5 study. Which of these identities are easy for members to understand and live out? Which of them are harder?

Ask members to share how they used the Day 6 and 7 reflections to deepen their understanding about God's refuge and applying that understanding in their lives.

—— WEEK THREE: A REFUGE OF HUMILITY

Invite members to join you in the neck exercise from Day 1. Ask members to share thoughts about being stiff-necked.

Jesus confronted pride and hypocrisy in the Pharisees. Why do some religious leaders tend to become hypocritical? How can we identify and eliminate hypocrisy in our lives?

How did comparing Cain and Hannah's stories connect to the comparison conflict? Ask members who are willing to share personal experiences.

Ask members to talk about Day 1's survey on personal pride. How did 2 Chronicles 7:14 help in confronting and conquering pride?

Review the cautionary tales from Day 5. How can we learn from these non-examples of humility? How can we choose God's refuge of humility over pride?

Ask members to share how they used the Day 6 and 7 reflections to deepen their understanding about God's refuge and applying that understanding in their lives.

—— WEEK FOUR: A REFUGE OF HEALING

Discuss David's parenting style. How did he impact the dysfunction of his family? How can the activities listed at the end of Day 1 help in processing pain caused by fractured families?

Naomi, Ruth, and the father of the prodigal son experienced grief and loss. How does the way we handle grief and loss reveal our dependence on God? How can we process the pain of grief and loss in healthy ways?

Ask a volunteer to read Psalm 34:18-19. Encourage members to share how God has provided a refuge of healing when trauma occurred. Ask another volunteer to read Joel 2:25-26. How has God repaid "the years the locusts have eaten?"

Eli the priest tried to fix his sons by not holding them accountable for their sins. How can we help others without becoming "fixers?"

"Pain is a gift that none of us want and yet none of us can do without." How can pain be a gift? Encourage members to share personal experiences.

Ask members to share how they used the Day 6 and 7 reflections to deepen their understanding about God's refuge and applying that understanding in their lives.

—— WEEK FIVE: A REFUGE OF MERCY

Ask members to share the synonyms for mercy they recorded and their responses to the merciful actions survey. How has God shown mercy, and how are we reflecting His mercy?

Review God's mercy toward Adam and Eve, Cain, and David. Encourage members to share their "but God" experiences.

Ask a volunteer to read Romans 8:1-2. Lead a discussion about how we deal with sin without self-condemnation.

Encourage members to share their responses to the 13 attributes of God's mercy from the Talmud. Ask members to share their ideas about empathy versus sympathy and examples of how they have given or received it.

How did God show grace to Noah and Jehoiachin? Discuss what it means to put aside our prison clothes and embrace God's refuge of mercy.

Ask members to share how they used the Day 6 and 7 reflections to deepen their understanding about God's refuge and applying that understanding in their lives.

—— WEEK SIX: A REFUGE OF FORGIVENESS

Lead a discussion about the desire for revenge. How can this desire hurt us? How does knowing God's love help us counteract vengeful desires? How do we deal with anger? How does the fermented wine illustration relate to bitterness?

How did King Saul play the "blame game" and how was that different than David? Review the questions and answers from Romans 8:31-39. How can we live as victors rather than victims?

Review the practice of forgiveness from Day 4. Encourage members to share their experiences with giving and receiving forgiveness that connect to these practices.

Encourage members to share their responses from analyzing the Sermon on the Mount from Day 5. How can your First Place for Health group members support each other in developing kingdom characteristics and embracing God's refuge of forgiveness?

Ask members to share how they used the Day 6 and 7 reflections to deepen their understanding about God's refuge and applying that understanding in their lives.

—— WEEK SEVEN: A REFUGE OF ACCEPTANCE

Discuss how the world judges people by their appearances. How does God view us? How is this different than the world?

Encourage members to share their thoughts on a positive body image. How does one's body image affect one's self-care and connectedness to God?

Review 1 Corinthians 13:4-7 and discuss how these verses teach us how to love ourselves in godly ways. How does denying ourselves for Christ's sake relate to self-love?

Lead a discussion about the difference between reproach and regret. Why is forgiving ourselves important to our fitness journey?

Review the story in John 8:2-11. How does Jesus rebuke condemnation and teach us to love ourselves in God's refuge of acceptance? Encourage members to share their deliverance experiences.

Ask members to share how they used the Day 6 and 7 reflections to deepen their understanding about God's refuge and applying that understanding in their lives.

—— WEEK EIGHT: A REFUGE OF JOY

Review the lessons from Elijah in Day 1's lesson. Ask members to share how these lessons connect to their fitness journeys.

Recount Elijah's experience in 1 Kings 18:41-46. How do the three lessons from this story relate to a refuge of joy? Encourage members to share how God is developing humility, patience, and strength in them.

Discuss how Elijah succumbed to pride after the Mount Carmel victory. How is pride a danger, and how can we avoid it after we experience a victory?

Ask members to share how God has spoken to them in either dramatic or quiet ways. How do these experiences reflect a refuge of joy?

Encourage members to share what they experienced after being on a mountaintop with God. How does the phrase "be strong and courageous" resonate?

Ask members to share how they used the Day 6 and 7 reflections to deepen their understanding about God's refuge and applying that understanding in their lives.

—— WEEK NINE: TIME TO CELEBRATE

As your class members reflect on each week's content, help them remember the ways strength has risen because of following Christ fully in each area of life. Ask: What have you learned in this study that has made you stronger?

FIRST PLACE FOR HEALTH
JUMP START MENUS

All recipe and menu nutritional information was determined using the MasterCook software, a program that accesses a database containing more than 6,000 food items prepared using the United States Department of Agriculture (USDA) publications and information from food manufacturers. As with any nutritional program, MasterCook calculates the nutritional values of the recipes based on ingredients. Nutrition may vary due to how the food is prepared, where the food comes from, soil content, season, ripeness, processing and method of preparation. For these reasons, please use the recipes and menu plans as approximate guides. As always, consult your physician and/or a registered dietitian before starting a weight-loss program.

For those who need more calories,
add the following to the 1,400–1,500 calorie plan:

1,500-1,600 calories:	1 oz.-eq of protein, 1 oz.-eq. grains, ½ cup vegetables, 1 tsp. healthy oils
1,700-1,800 calories:	1½ oz.-eq. of protein, 2 oz.-eq. grains, 1 cup of vegetables, 1 tsp. healthy oils
1,900-2,000 calories:	2 oz.-eq. of protein, 2 oz.-eq. of grains, 1 cup vegetables, ½ cup fruit, 1 tsp. healthy oils
2,100-2,200 calories:	3 oz.-eq. of protein, 3 oz.-eq. grains, 1½ cup vegetables, ½ cup fruit, 2 tsp. healthy oils
2,300-2,400 calories:	4 oz.-eq. of protein, 4 oz.-eq. of grains, 2 cups vegetables 3 cups frit, 3 tsp. healthy oils

DAY 1 | BREAKFAST

Hash Brown Egg Cups

2 medium russet potatoes (about 2 cups shredded)
1/2 cup shredded cheese
Salt and ground pepper
Nonstick cooking spray
4-6 eggs
Salt and pepper to taste
Parsley for serving

Preheat the oven to 350° F. Grease a 6-cup muffin pan generously with cooking spray. Peel the potatoes, then use a large box grater to grate the uncooked potatoes. Transfer the grated potatoes to a colander and rinse until the water runs clear. Dry the potatoes thoroughly with paper towels. Divide the hash browns evenly between the muffin cups. Use your fingers to pack them tightly and shape them into nests or press down with a small measuring cup. Season with salt and pepper. Spray again with cooking spray.

Bake until golden and the edges start to brown, about 15 to 20 minutes. Then remove cups from oven. Whisk the four eggs together and season with salt and pepper. You can add any toppings into the mixture. Carefully divide the eggs between the six egg cups and sprinkle shredded cheese on top. Bake until the egg whites set, about 12-15 minutes. Cool for 5 minutes before removing from pan. Serves 6

Nutritional Information: Calories: 126; 13g Carbohydrates; 7g Protein 5g; Fat; 116mg Cholesterol; 109mg Sodium: 109mg; 1g Fiber

DAY 1 | LUNCH

Black Bean Salad

- 2 cups chopped romaine lettuce
- 1 avocado, chopped
- 1 medium tomato, chopped
- ½ cup canned black beans, rinsed
- 2 tbsp. diced green onion
- 1 tbsp. diced fresh cilantro
- 1 tbsp. olive oil
- 2 tsp lime juice
- ¼ tsp. lime zest
- ¼ tsp. salt
- ½ tsp. ground black pepper

In a large bowl, toss together lettuce, avocado, tomato, beans, green onion and cilantro. In a small bowl, mix olive oil, lime juice, lime zest, salt and pepper. Pour dressing over salad and toss well to coat. Serve with baked tortilla chips. Serves 2

Nutritional Information: 247 calories; 17g fat; 6g protein; 20g carbohydrate; 9g dietary fiber; 311 mg sodium.

DAY 1 | DINNER

Grilled Chicken & Polenta with Blackberry Salsa

1 tablespoon plus 1 teaspoon canola oil, divided
1 tablespoon ground cumin
1 teaspoon kosher salt, divided
3/4 teaspoon freshly ground pepper
1 16- to 18-ounce tube prepared plain polenta
1 pound boneless, skinless chicken breast, trimmed
2 nectarines, halved and pitted
1 pint blackberries, coarsely chopped
2 tablespoons chopped fresh cilantro
1 tablespoon lime juice
Hot sauce to taste

Preheat grill to medium-high. Combine 1 tablespoon oil, cumin, 3/4 teaspoon salt and pepper in a small bowl. Rub 1 teaspoon of the mixture all over polenta. Rub the rest into both sides of chicken. Cut the polenta crosswise into 8 slices. Rub the cut sides of nectarine halves with the remaining 1 teaspoon oil. Oil the grill rack (see Tip). Place the chicken, polenta slices and nectarines on the grill. Grill the polenta until hot and slightly charred, 3 to 4 minutes per side. Transfer to a plate and keep warm. Grill the nectarines, turning occasionally, until tender, 6 to 8 minutes total. Grill the chicken, until cooked through and no longer pink in the middle, 6 to 8 minutes per side. Transfer the chicken and nectarines to a cutting board. Coarsely chop the nectarines. Let the chicken rest for 5 minutes, then thinly slice. While the chicken rests, combine the chopped nectarines, blackberries, cilantro, lime juice, hot sauce and the remaining 1/4 teaspoon salt in a medium bowl. Layer the polenta, chicken and fruit salsa on 4 plates and serve. Serves 4

Nutritional Information: 317 calories; 8 g fat; 63 mg cholesterol; 34 g carbohydrate; 27 g protein; 6 g fiber; 694 mg sodium; 458 mg potassium.

DAY 2 | BREAKFAST

Egg Muffins with Broccoli

9 large eggs
1/4 cup feta
1/4 cup part-skim mozzarella cheese, shredded
1 tbsp garlic powder
1/2 tsp salt
1/2 tsp black pepper
1/8 tsp red pepper flakes
1 cup quinoa cooked
2 cups broccoli
1/2 cup parsley
2 green onion sprigs chopped
Cooking spray

Preheat oven to 350° F. Place muffin liners into a 12-muffin tin and spray with cooking spray. In large mixing bowl, whisk eggs until well mixed. Add feta, mozzarella, garlic powder, salt, pepper, red pepper flakes and stir to combine. Add quinoa, broccoli, parsley and green onions, mix. Fill each muffin with egg mixture 3/4 full and sprinkle with extra mozzarella cheese on top (optional). Bake for 20 mins. Remove and let cool about 10 minutes.

Store: Refrigerate in an airtight container for up to 5 days. Reheat in microwave.

Freeze: Keep in an airtight container for up to 3 months. Defrost in a microwave or thaw on a counter. Serves 12

Nutritional Information: 93 Calories; 6g Carbohydrate; 7g Protein; 5g Fat; 127mg Cholesterol; 1g Fiber; 199mg Sodium

DAY 2 | LUNCH

Fresh Tomato Soup

- 2 cups fat-free, low-sodium chicken broth
- 1 cup chopped onion
- ¾ cup chopped celery
- 1 tbsp. thinly sliced fresh basil
- 1 tbsp. tomato paste
- 2 lbs. roma tomatoes, cut into wedges
- ½ tsp. salt
- ¼ tsp. freshly ground black pepper
- 6 tbsp. plain lowfat yogurt
- 3 tbsp. thinly sliced fresh basil

Combine chicken broth, onion, celery, basil, tomato paste and tomatoes in a large saucepan and bring to a boil. Reduce heat and simmer 30 minutes. Place half of the tomato mixture in a blender. Vent blender lid to allow steam to escape and secure the blender lid on the blender. Place a clean towel over the opening in the blender lid to avoid splatters and blend until smooth. Pour the mixture into a large bowl and repeat the procedure with the remaining tomato mixture. Stir in salt and pepper. Ladle ¾ cup soup into each of 6 bowls and top each serving with 1 tablespoon yogurt and 1½ teaspoons basil. Serving suggestion: Serve with ½ turkey sandwich on whole-grain bread with light mayo or Dijon mustard, lettuce and tomato. Serves 6.

Nutritional Information: 58 calories; 1g fat; 3g protein; 11g carbohydrate; 3g dietary fiber; 1mg cholesterol; 382mg sodium.

DAY 2 | DINNER

Tilapia & Vegetable Packets

- 1 cup quartered cherry or grape tomatoes
- 1 cup diced summer squash
- 1 cup thinly sliced red onion
- 12 green beans, trimmed and cut into 1-inch pieces
- 1/4 cup pitted and coarsely chopped black olives
- 2 tablespoons lemon juice
- 1 tablespoon chopped fresh oregano
- 1 tablespoon extra-virgin olive oil
- 1 teaspoon capers, rinsed
- 1/2 teaspoon salt, divided
- 1/2 teaspoon freshly ground pepper, divided
- 1 pound tilapia fillets, cut into 4 equal portions

Preheat grill to medium. Combine tomatoes, squash, onion, green beans, olives, lemon juice, oregano, oil, capers, 1/4 teaspoon salt and 1/4 teaspoon pepper in a large bowl. To make a packet, lay two 20-inch sheets of foil on top of each other. Generously coat the top piece with cooking spray. Place one portion of tilapia in the center of the foil. Sprinkle with some of the remaining 1/4 teaspoon salt and pepper, then top with 3/4 cup of the vegetable mixture. Bring the short ends of the foil together, leaving enough room in the packet for steam to gather and cook the food. Fold the foil over and pinch to seal. Pinch seams together along the sides. Make sure all the seams are tightly sealed to keep steam from escaping. Repeat with more foil, cooking spray and the remaining fish, salt, pepper and vegetables. Grill the packets until the fish is cooked through and the vegetables are just tender, about 5 minutes. To serve, carefully open both ends of the packets and allow the steam to escape. Slide the contents onto plates.

Oven Variation: Preheat oven to 425° F. Place green beans in a microwavable bowl with 1 tablespoon water. Cover and microwave on High until the beans are just beginning to cook, about 30 seconds. Drain and add to the other vegetables. Assemble packets as listed above. Bake the packets directly on an oven rack until the tilapia is cooked through and the vegetables are just tender, about 20 minutes.

Nutritional Information: Per serving: 181 calories; 7 g fat; 57 mg cholesterol; 8 g carbohydrate; 24 g protein; 2 g fiber; 435 mg sodium

DAY 3 | BREAKFAST

Baked Oatmeal

2 cups rolled oats
½ cup pecan pieces
1 teaspoon baking powder
1 ½ teaspoons cinnamon
½ teaspoon allspice
½ teaspoon kosher salt
1 apple, cut into small cubes (can substitute 1 cup blueberries, raspberries, raisins, or dried cranberries)
1 large egg
2 cups low-fat milk
⅓ cup pure maple syrup, plus 1 tablespoon for drizzling
2 teaspoons vanilla extract
1 tablespoon salted butter

Preheat the oven to 375° F. Butter an 8 x 8" pan. In medium bowl, mix the rolled oats, pecan pieces, baking powder, cinnamon, allspice, and kosher salt. Place into prepared pan and spread evenly. Add diced apple in even layer on top of oat mixture. Whisk the egg, then add milk, maple syrup, and vanilla. Drizzle milk mixture over the oats and apples. Use a fork to lightly stir so it is evenly incorporated. Bake 40 to 45 minutes, or until golden and oat mixture has set. Remove from oven and allow to cool for 10 minutes. Melt butter with the remaining 1 tablespoon maple syrup. Drizzle the butter evenly over the top and serve. Store leftovers refrigerated for up to 1 week or freeze for up to 3 months. Serves 8

Nutritional Information: 213 Calories; 7g Fat; 30g Carbohydrate; 6.1g Protein; 3.5g Fiber

DAY 3 | LUNCH

BLT Salad

¼ cup fat-free mayonnaise
3 tbsp. thinly sliced green onions
3 tbsp. reduced-fat sour cream
2 tsp. whole-grain Dijon mustard
½ tsp. freshly ground black pepper
¼ tsp. grated lemon rind
8 hard-cooked large eggs
8 (1½-oz.) slices firm sandwich bread, toasted
4 center-cut bacon slices, cooked and cut in half crosswise
8 (¼-inch-thick) slices tomato
4 large lettuce leaves

Combine mayonnaise, onions, sour cream, Dijon mustard, pepper and lemon rind in a medium bowl, stirring well. Cut 2 eggs in half lengthwise, and reserve the yolks for another use. Coarsely chop the remaining egg whites and whole eggs. Add eggs to the mayonnaise mixture and stir gently to combine. Next, arrange 4 bread slices on a cutting board or work surface. Top each bread slice with ½ cup of the egg mixture, 2 bacon pieces, 2 tomato slices, 1 lettuce leaf and 1 bread slice. Serves 4.

Nutritional Information: 371 calories; 11.7g fat; 22g protein; 44g carbohydrate; 2g dietary fiber; 329mg cholesterol; 892mg sodium.

DAY 3 | DINNER

Roasted Chicken with Butternut Squash

2 tbsp. minced garlic
1 tsp. salt
3/4 tsp. freshly ground black pepper
1/2 teaspoon dried sage
1 (3 1/2-pound) roasting chicken
nonstick cooking spray
12 oz. red potatoes, cut into wedges
1 1/2 cups cubed peeled butternut squash
2 tbsp. butter, melted

Preheat oven to 400° F. Combine 1 1/2 tablespoons garlic, 1/2 teaspoon salt, 1/2 teaspoon pepper and sage in a small bowl. Remove and discard giblets and neck from chicken. Starting at neck cavity, loosen skin from breast and drumsticks by inserting fingers, gently pushing between skin and meat. Lift wing tips up and over back, and then tuck under chicken. Rub the garlic mixture under loosened skin. Place chicken, breast side up, on rack of a broiler pan coated with nonstick cooking spray. Place rack in a broiler pan. Combine potatoes, squash, butter, 1/2 teaspoons garlic, 1/2 teaspoon salt and 1/4 teaspoon pepper. Arrange vegetable mixture around chicken. Bake at 400° for 1 hour or until a thermometer inserted into meaty part of thigh registers 165°. Let stand for 10 minutes. Discard skin. Serves 4

Nutritional Information: 399 calories; 12g fat; 43.8g protein; 25.9g carbohydrate; 3.4g fiber; 147mg cholesterol; 791mg sodium

DAY 4 | BREAKFAST

Banana Oatmeal Bake

1 egg
¼ cup peanut butter
¼ cup pure maple syrup
1 cup mashed overripe banana (2 large or 3 medium)
1 ½ cups grated zucchini (1 medium zucchini)
½ cup low fat milk
1 tsp vanilla extract
3 cups old-fashioned oats
1 tbsp baking powder
1 tsp cinnamon
½ tsp fine sea salt

Preheat oven to 375° F. Spray a muffin tin with cooking spray. Mix mashed banana, grated zucchini, milk, vanilla extract, peanut butter, maple syrup, and egg, stirring to combine.

Add oats, baking powder, cinnamon, salt, and add-ins of choice (see below). Stir until just combined. Spoon mixture into muffin cups, filling to the top. Makes 16 muffins. Bake for about 26 minutes, or until a fork comes out clean. Cool on wire rack. Store cooled oatmeal cups in an air-tight container in the refrigerator for up to one week or freeze for up to 3 months. Serves 16

Optional add-ins: ¼ cup chocolate chips and/or nuts.

Nutritional Information: 112 Calories; 2.5g Fat; 12mg Cholesterol; 4g Protein; 2.6g Fiber; 80mg Sodium

DAY 4 | LUNCH

Barbecue Chicken Sandwich

½ cup shredded cooked chicken
¼ cup shredded carrots
2 tbsp. barbecue sauce
2 tsp. light Ranch dressing
1 small whole-wheat sandwich bun
1 leaf romaine lettuce

Combine chicken, carrots and barbecue sauce in a bowl. Spread Ranch dressing on the bun and top with the chicken mixture and lettuce. Serve with baked chips. Serves 1

Nutritional Information: 323 calories; 8g fat; 26g protein; 37g carbohydrates; 4g fiber; 62mg cholesterol; 729mg sodium.

DAY 4 | DINNER

Fish Fillets Florentine

    4 5-oz. tilapia fillets
    1/4 tsp. lemon-pepper seasoning
    1 10-oz. frozen creamed spinach, thawed
    1/4 cup fine dry Italian bread crumbs
    1/4 cup shredded 2% cheddar cheese
    nonstick cooking spray

Preheat oven to 400° F. Season fillets with lemon-pepper seasoning, arrange on a baking sheet coated with nonstick cooking spray, and set aside. In a small bowl, combine thawed spinach with bread crumbs. Spoon mixture evenly over the fillets and bake for 15 minutes or until fish flakes easily. Top each fillet with 1 tablespoon cheese and bake for 1 to 2 minutes more or until cheese is melted. Serves 4.

Nutritional Information: 283 calories; 12g fat; 28g protein; 10g carbohydrate; 1g fiber; 82mg cholesterol; 590mg sodium

DAY 5 | BREAKFAST

Cereal Sundae

¾ cups bran flakes
6 oz. light lemon or vanilla yogurt
2 tbsp. walnuts

Top yogurt with bran flakes and walnuts. Serves 1.

Nutritional Information: 298 calories; 10g fat; 15g protein; 45g carbohydrate; 8g fiber; 2mg cholesterol; 358mg sodium.

DAY 5 | LUNCH

Turkey Sandwich with Lemon Mayo

1 tsp. grated lemon peel
1 tbsp. low-fat mayonnaise
2 slices whole-grain bread
1 cup loosely packed baby spinach leaves
2 oz. turkey breast, sliced
1 small tomato, sliced

Stir the grated lemon peel into the mayonnaise and spread on both slices of bread. On one slice of the bread, alternately layer spinach leaves, turkey and tomato, starting and ending with spinach. Top with the second bread slice. Serves 1.

Nutritional Information: 300 calories; 7g fat; 26g protein; 33g carbohydrate; 13g fiber; 57mg cholesterol; 320mg sodium.

DAY 5 | DINNER

Crispy Fish Taco Bowls

1 pound white fish, such as cod, cut into 2-inch pieces
½ cup light mayonnaise, divided
¾ cup panko breadcrumbs
¼ cup light sour cream
2 tablespoons adobo sauce
2 tablespoons lime juice
Pinch of salt plus 1/4 teaspoon, divided
¼ teaspoon ground pepper
2 cups cooked brown rice
2 cups shredded cabbage
1 cup thinly sliced radishes
Fresh cilantro

Preheat oven to 475° F. Place a wire rack on a rimmed baking sheet; coat with cooking spray. Coat fish with 1/4 cup mayonnaise. Place panko in a shallow dish and roll the fish in it until fully coated. Transfer to wire rack. Bake the fish until crispy and cooked through, 8 to 12 minutes, depending on thickness. Meanwhile, mix the remaining 1/4 cup mayonnaise, sour cream, adobo sauce, lime juice and pinch of salt in a small bowl. Sprinkle the fish with the remaining 1/4 teaspoon salt and pepper. Divide rice among 4 bowls and top with the fish, cabbage, radishes, the sauce and cilantro, if desired. Serves 4

Nutritional Information: 325 calories; 10g protein; 42g carbohydrates; 3g fiber; 25g fat 53mg cholesterol 63mg; 738mg sodium

DAY 6 | BREAKFAST

Waffles with Blueberry Maple Syrup

1/3 cup frozen blueberries
2 tsp. maple syrup
2 whole-grain waffles
1 tbsp. pecans

Microwave blueberries and syrup together for 2 to 3 minutes, until berries are thawed.

Toast the waffles, top with warm blueberry syrup, and sprinkle with pecans. Serves 1.

Nutritional Information: 305 calories; 14g fat; 8g protein; 41g carbohydrate; 4g dietary fiber

DAY 6 | LUNCH

Chicken and Spinach Salad

2 cups cooked chicken, cubed
6 cup packed fresh spinach, torn into bite-sized pieces
2 oranges, peeled and cut into chunks
2 cups fresh strawberries, sliced

Orange-Poppy Dressing
2 tablespoon red wine vinegar
3 tablespoon orange juice
1 1/2 tablespoon canola oil
1/4 teaspoon dry mustard
1/4 teaspoon poppy seeds

In large bowl, combine chicken, spinach, oranges and strawberries. In separate bowl, combine all ingredients for Orange-Poppy Dressing, mix well. Toss dressing with salad and mix well to coat. Serves 4.

Nutritional Information: 307 Calories; 9g Fat; 26g Protein; 30g Carbohydrate; 6g Fiber; 60mg Cholesterol; 240mg Sodium

DAY 6 | DINNER

Sheet Pan Balsamic Chicken

    3 chicken breasts, diced into small pieces
    1 carrot, chopped
    1 zucchini, chopped
    1/2 cup Brussels sprouts, sliced in half
    1 red pepper, chopped
    2 tbsp balsamic vinegar
    1 tbsp olive oil
    1 tbsp Dijon mustard
    4 cloves garlic minced
    2 tsp Italian seasoning
    1/2 tsp each salt & pepper

Preheat oven to 450° F. Toss all ingredients together in large bowl and place on parchment-lined baking sheet. Bake for 15 minutes, stirring halfway through, until veggies and chicken are fully cooked. Divide into four bowls. Serves 4

Nutritional Information: 263 Calories; 8g Carbohydrates; 31g Protein; 12g Fat; 83mg Cholesterol; 3g Fiber; 467mg Sodium

DAY 7 | BREAKFAST

Spinach & Bacon Omelet

    1 egg plus 2 egg whites
    2 slices cooked turkey bacon, crumbled
    1 cup baby spinach
    1 slice whole-grain toast
    1 tsp. butter
    nonstick cooking spray

Whisk together eggs, bacon and spinach. Coat a skillet with nonstick cooking spray. Cook the egg mixture and serve with toast and butter. Serves 1

Nutritional Information: 308 calories; 16g fat, 24g protein; 16g carbohydrate, 2g fiber

DAY 7 | LUNCH

Grilled Goat Cheese Sandwich

2 teaspoons honey
1/4 teaspoon grated lemon rind
1 (4-ounce) package goat cheese
8 (1-ounce) slices cinnamon-raisin bread
2 tablespoons fig preserves
2 teaspoons thinly sliced fresh basil
Cooking spray
1 teaspoon powdered sugar

Combine first 3 ingredients, stirring until well blended. Spread 1 tablespoon goat cheese mixture on each of 4 bread slices; top each slice with 1 1/2 teaspoons preserves and 1/2 teaspoon basil. Top with remaining bread slices. Lightly coat outside of bread with cooking spray. Heat a large nonstick skillet over medium heat. Add 2 sandwiches to pan. Place a cast-iron or heavy skillet on top of sandwiches; press gently to flatten. Cook 3 minutes on each side or until bread is lightly toasted (leave cast-iron skillet on sandwiches while they cook). Repeat with remaining sandwiches. Sprinkle with sugar. Serves 4

Nutritional Information: 288 Calories; 11g Fat; 13g Protein; 34g Carbohydrate; 2g Fiber; 30mg Cholesterol; 240mg Sodium

DAY 7 | DINNER

Salmon Tacos with Pineapple Salsa

1 (1 pound) salmon fillet
1 teaspoon chili powder
¾ teaspoon salt, divided
1 tablespoon plus 1 teaspoon extra-virgin olive oil, divided
1 (9 ounce) package coleslaw mix (5 cups)
½ lime, juiced
8 (6 inch) corn tortillas, warmed
¾ cup purchased pineapple salsa
Chopped fresh cilantro, for garnish
Hot sauce for serving

Arrange oven rack in upper third of oven so salmon will be 2 to 3 inches below heat source. Preheat broiler to high. Line a baking sheet with foil. Lay salmon on the foil, skin-side down. Broil, rotating the pan from front to back once, until the salmon is starting to brown, is opaque on the sides and the thinner parts of the fillet are sizzling, 5 to 8 minutes, depending on thickness. Sprinkle the salmon with chili powder and 1/4 teaspoon salt. Drizzle with 1 teaspoon oil and brush with a heatproof brush to moisten the spices. Return to the oven and continue broiling until the salmon just flakes and the spices are browned, 1 to 2 minutes more. Meanwhile, toss coleslaw mix with lime juice, the remaining 1 tablespoon oil and the remaining 1/2 teaspoon salt. Flake the salmon, discarding skin. Divide the salmon among tortillas and top with salsa. Serve with the coleslaw and garnish with cilantro and hot sauce, if desired. Serves 4 (2 tacos per serving)

Nutritional Information: 320 calories; 25g protein; 29g carbohydrates; 3.5g fiber; 10.5g fat 53mg cholesterol; 592mg sodium

STEPS FOR SPIRITUAL GROWTH

—— GOD'S WORD FOR YOUR LIFE

I have hidden your word in my heart that I might not sin against you.

Psalm 119:11

As you begin to make decisions based on what God's Word teaches you, you will want to memorize what He has promised to those who trust and follow Him. Second Peter 1:3 tells us that God "has given us everything we need for life and godliness through our knowledge of him" (emphasis added). The Bible provides instruction and encouragement for any area of life in which you may be struggling. If you are dealing with a particular emotion or traumatic life event—fear, discouragement, stress, financial upset, the death of a loved one, a relationship difficulty—you can search through a Bible concordance for Scripture passages that deal with that particular situation. Scripture provides great comfort to those who memorize it.

One of the promises of knowing and obeying God's Word is that it gives you wisdom, insight, and understanding above all worldly knowledge (see Psalm 119:97–104). Psalm 119:129–130 says, "Your statutes are wonderful; therefore I obey them. The unfolding of your words gives light; it gives understanding to the simple." Now that's a precious promise about guidance for life!

The Value of Scripture Memory

Scripture memory is an important part of the Christian life. There are four key reasons to memorize Scripture:

1. **TO HANDLE DIFFICULT SITUATIONS.** A heartfelt knowledge of God's Word will equip you to handle any situation that you might face. Declaring such truth as, "I can do everything through Christ" (see Philippians 4:13) and "he will never leave me or forsake me" (see Hebrews 13:5) will enable you to walk through situations with peace and courage.

2. **TO OVERCOME TEMPTATION.** Luke 4:1–13 describes how Jesus used Scripture to overcome His temptations in the desert (see also Matthew 4:1-11). Knowledge of Scripture and the strength that comes with the ability to use it are important parts of putting on the full armor of God in preparation for spiritual warfare (see Ephesians 6:10–18).

3. **TO GET GUIDANCE.** Psalm 119:105 states the Word of God "is a lamp to my feet and a light for my path." You learn to hide God's Word in your heart so His light will direct your decisions and actions throughout your day.

4. **TO TRANSFORM YOUR MIND.** "Do not conform any longer to the pattern of this world, but be transformed by the renewing of your mind" (Romans 12:2). Scripture memory allows you to replace a lie with the truth of God's Word. When Scripture becomes firmly settled in your memory, not only will your thoughts connect with God's thoughts, but you will also be able to honor God with small everyday decisions as well as big life-impacting ones. Scripture memorization is the key to making a permanent lifestyle change in your thought patterns, which brings balance to every other area of your life.

Scripture Memory Tips

- Write the verse down, saying it aloud as you write it.
- Read verses before and after the memory verse to get its context.
- Read the verse several times, emphasizing a different word each time.
- Connect the Scripture reference to the first few words.
- Locate patterns, phrases, or keywords.
- Apply the Scripture to circumstances you are now experiencing.
- Pray the verse, making it personal to your life and inserting your name as the recipient of the promise or teaching. (Try that with 1 Corinthians 10:13, inserting "me" and "I" for "you.")
- Review the verse every day until it becomes second nature to think those words whenever your circumstances match its message. The Holy Spirit will bring the verse to mind when you need it most if you decide to plant it in your memory.

Scripture Memorization Made Easy!

What is your learning style? Do you learn by hearing, by sight, or by doing?

If you learn by hearing—if you are an auditory learner—singing the Scripture memory verses, reading them aloud, or recording them and listening to your recording will be very helpful in the memorization process.

If you are a visual learner, writing the verses and repeatedly reading through them will cement them in your mind.

If you learn by doing—if you are a tactile learner—creating motions for the words or using sign language will enable you to more easily recall the verse.

After determining your learning style, link your Scripture memory with a daily task, such as driving to work, walking on a treadmill, or eating lunch. Use these daily tasks as opportunities to memorize and review your verses.

Meals at home or out with friends can be used as a time to share the verse you are memorizing with those at your table. You could close your personal email messages by typing in your weekly memory verse. Or why not say your memory verse every time you brush your teeth or put on your shoes?

The purpose of Scripture memorization is to be able to apply God's words to your life. If you memorize Scripture using methods that connect with your particular learning style, you will find it easier to hide God's Word in your heart.

──ESTABLISHING A QUIET TIME

Like all other components of the First Place for Health program, developing a live relationship with God is not a random act. You must intentionally seek God if you are to find Him! It's not that God plays hide-and-seek with you. He is always available to you. He invites you to come boldly into His presence. He reveals Himself to you in the pages of the Bible. And once you decide to earnestly seek Him, you are sure to find Him! When you delight in Him, your gracious God will give you the desires of your heart. Spending time getting to know God involves four basic elements: a priority, a plan, a place, and practice.

A Priority

You can successfully establish a quiet time with God by making this meeting a daily priority. This may require carving out time in your day so you have time and space for this new relationship you are cultivating. Often this will mean eliminating less important things so you will have time and space to meet with God. When speaking about Jesus, John the Baptist said, "He must become greater; I must become less" (John 3:30). You will undoubtedly find that to be true as well. What might you need to eliminate from your current schedule so that spending quality time with God can become a priority?

A Plan

Having made quiet time a priority, you will want to come up with a plan. This plan will include the time you have set aside to spend with God and a general outline of how you will spend your time in God's presence.

Elements you should consider incorporating into your quiet time include:

- Singing a song of praise
- Reading a daily selection in a devotional book or reading a psalm
- Using a systematic Scripture reading plan so you will be exposed to the whole truth of God's Word
- Completing your First Place for Health Bible study for that day
- Praying—silent, spoken, and written prayer
- Writing in your spiritual journal.

You will also want to make a list of the materials you will need to make your encounter with God more meaningful:

- A Bible
- Your First Place for Health Bible study
- Your prayer journal
- A pen and/or pencil
- A devotional book
- A Bible concordance
- A college-level dictionary
- A box of tissues (tears—both of sadness and joy—are often part of our quiet time with God!)

Think of how you would plan an important business meeting or social event, and then transfer that knowledge to your meeting time with God.

A Place

Having formulated a meeting-with-God plan, you will next need to create a meeting-with-God place. Of course, God is always with you; however, in order to have quality devotional time with Him, it is desirable that you find a comfortable meeting place. You will want to select a spot that is quiet and as distraction-free as possible. Meeting with God in the same place on a regular basis will help you remember what you are there for: to have an encounter with the true and living God!

Having selected the place, put the materials you have determined to use in your quiet time into a basket or on a nearby table or shelf. Now take the time to establish your personal quiet time with God. Tailor your quiet time to fit your needs—and the time you have allotted to spend with God. Although many people elect to meet with God early in the morning, for others afternoon or evening is best. There is no hard-and-fast rule about when your quiet time should be—the only essential thing is that you establish a quiet time!

Start with a small amount of time that you know you can devote yourself to daily. You can be confident that as you consistently spend time with God each day, the amount of time you can spend will increase as you are ready for the next level of your walk with God.

I will meet with God from _____ to _____ daily.

I plan to use that time with God to _____

Supplies I will need to assemble include _____

My meeting place with God will be _____

Practice

After you have chosen the time and place to meet God each day and you have assembled your supplies, there are four easy steps for having a fruitful and worshipful time with the Lord.

STEP 1: *Clear Your Heart and Mind*

"Be still, and know that I am God" (Psalm 46:10). Begin your quiet time by reading the daily Bible selection from a devotional guide or a psalm. If you are new in your Christian walk, an excellent devotional guide to use is *Streams in the Desert* by L.B. Cowman. More mature Christians might benefit from *My Utmost for His Highest* by Oswald Chambers. Of course, you can use any devotional that has a strong emphasis on Scripture and prayer.

STEP 2: Read and Interact with Scripture

"I have hidden your word in my heart that I might not sin against you" (Psalm 119:11). As you open your Bible, ask the Holy Spirit to reveal something He knows you need for this day through the reading of His Word. Always try to find a nugget to encourage or direct you through the day. As you read the passage, pay special attention to the words and phrases the Holy Spirit brings to your attention. Some words may seem to resonate in your soul. You will want to spend time meditating on the passage, asking God what lesson He is teaching you.

After reading the Scripture passage over several times, ask yourself the following questions:

- In light of what I have read today, is there something I must now do? (Confess a sin? Claim a promise? Follow an example? Obey a command? Avoid a situation?)
- How should I respond to what I've read today?

STEP 3: Pray

"Be clear minded and self-controlled so that you can pray" (1 Peter 4:7). Spend time conversing with the Lord in prayer. Prayer is such an important part of First Place for Health that there is an entire section in this member's guide devoted to the practice of prayer.

STEP 4: Praise

"Praise the LORD, O my soul, and forget not all his benefits" (Psalm 103:2). End your quiet time with a time of praise. Be sure to thank the Lord of heaven and warmth for choosing to spend time with you!

—— SHARING YOUR FAITH

Nothing is more effective in drawing someone to Jesus than sharing personal life experiences. People are more open to the good news of Jesus Christ when they see faith in action. Personal faith stories are simple and effective ways to share what Christ is doing in your life, because they show firsthand how Christ makes a difference.

Sharing your faith story has an added benefit: it builds you up in your faith, too! Is your experience in First Place for Health providing you opportunities to share with others what God is doing in your life? If you answered yes, then you have a personal faith story!

If you do not have a personal faith story, perhaps it is because you don't know Jesus Christ as your personal Lord and Savior. Read through "Steps to Becoming a Christian" (which is the next chapter) and begin today to give Christ first place in your life.

Creativity and preparation in using opportunities to share a word or story about Jesus is an important part of the Christian life. Is Jesus helping you in a special way? Are you achieving a level of success or peace that you haven't experienced in other attempts to lose weight, exercise regularly, or eat healthier? As people see you making changes and achieving success, they may ask you how you are doing it. How will—or do—you respond? Remember, your story is unique, and it may allow others to see what Christ is doing in your life. It may also help to bring Christ into the life of another person.

Personal Statements of Faith

First Place for Health gives you a great opportunity to communicate your faith and express what God is doing in your life. Be ready to use your own personal statement of faith whenever the opportunity presents itself. Personal statements of faith should be short and fit naturally into a conversation. They don't require or expect any action or response from the listener. The goal is not to get another person to change but simply to help you communicate who you are and what's important to you.

Here are some examples of short statements of faith that you might use when someone asks what you are doing to lose weight:

- "I've been meeting with a group at my church. We pray together, support each other, learn about nutrition, and study the Bible."
- "It's amazing how Bible study and prayer are helping me lose weight and eat healthier."
- "I've had a lot of support from a group I meet with at church."
- "I'm relying more on God to help me make changes in my lifestyle."

Begin keeping a list of your meaningful experiences as you go through the First Place for Health program. Also notice what is happening in the lives of others. Use the following questions to help you prepare short personal statements and stories of faith:

- What is God doing in your life physically, mentally, emotionally, and spiritually?
- How has your relationship with God changed? Is it more intimate or personal?
- How is prayer, Bible study, and/or the support of others helping you achieve your goals for a healthy weight and good nutrition?

Writing Your Personal Faith Story

Write a brief story about how God is working in your life through First Place for Health. Use your story to help you share with others what's happening in your life.

Use the following questions to help develop your story:

- Why did you join First Place for Health? What specific circumstances led you to a Christ-centered health and weight-loss program? What were you feeling when you joined?
- What was your relationship with Christ when you started First Place for Health? What is it now?
- Has your experience in First Place for Health changed your relationship with Christ? With yourself? With others?
- How has your relationship with Christ, prayer, Bible study, and group support made a difference in your life?
- What specific verse or passage of Scripture has made a difference in the way you view yourself or your relationship with Christ?
- What experiences have impacted your life since starting First Place for Health?
- In what ways is Christ working in your life today? In what ways is He meeting your needs?
- How has Christ worked in other members of your First Place for Health group?

Answer the above questions in a few sentences, and then use your answers to help you write your own short personal faith story.

MEMBER SURVEY

We would love to know more about you. Share this form with your leader.

Name _____   Birth date _____

Tell us about your family.

_____
_____
_____
_____

Would you like to receive more information   Yes   No
about our church?

What area of expertise would you be willing to share with our class?

_____
_____

Why did you join First Place for Health?

_____
_____

With notice, would you be willing to lead a Bible study   Yes   No
discussion one week?

Are you comfortable praying out loud? _____

Would you be willing to assist recording weights and/or   Yes   No
evaluating the Live It Trackers?

Any other comments:

_____
_____

PERSONAL WEIGHT AND MEASUREMENT RECORD

WEEK	WEIGHT	+ OR -	GOAL THIS SESSION	POUNDS TO GOAL
1				
2				
3				
4				
5				
6				
7				
8				
9				
10				
11				
12				

BEGINNING MEASUREMENTS

WAIST _____   HIPS _____   THIGHS _____   CHEST _____

ENDING MEASUREMENTS

WAIST _____   HIPS _____   THIGHS _____   CHEST _____

PRAYER PARTNER   WEEK 1

Since, then, you have been raised with Christ, set your hearts on things above,
where Christ is, seated at the right hand of God.
Colossians 3:1

Date: _____

Name: _____

Home Phone: _____

Cell Phone: _____

Email: _____

Personal Prayer Concerns

_____

_____

_____

_____

_____

_____

_____

_____

This form is for prayer requests that are personal to you and your journey in First Place for Health. Please complete and have it ready to turn in when you arrive at your group meeting.

PRAYER PARTNER　　　　　　　　　　　　WEEK 2

The Lord is a refuge for the oppressed, a stronghold
in times of trouble.
Psalm 9:9

Date: _____

Name: _____

Home Phone: _____

Cell Phone: _____

Email: _____

Personal Prayer Concerns

_____

_____

_____

_____

_____

_____

_____

_____

This form is for prayer requests that are personal to you and your journey in First Place for Health. Please complete and have it ready to turn in when you arrive at your group meeting.

PRAYER PARTNER   WEEK 3

Therefore, as it is written: "Let the one who boasts boast in the Lord."
1 Corinthians 1:31

Date: _____

Name: _____

Home Phone: _____

Cell Phone: _____

Email: _____

Personal Prayer Concerns

_____

_____

_____

_____

_____

_____

_____

This form is for prayer requests that are personal to you and your journey in First Place for Health. Please complete and have it ready to turn in when you arrive at your group meeting.

PRAYER PARTNER WEEK 4

He himself bore our sins in his body on the cross, so that we might die to sins and live for righteousness; "by his wounds you have been healed."
1 Peter 2:24

Date: _____

Name: _____

Home Phone: _____

Cell Phone: _____

Email: _____

Personal Prayer Concerns

_____

_____

_____

_____

_____

_____

_____

_____

This form is for prayer requests that are personal to you and your journey in First Place for Health. Please complete and have it ready to turn in when you arrive at your group meeting.

PRAYER PARTNER WEEK 5

The Lord is gracious and full of compassion, slow to anger and great in mercy. The Lord is good to all, and His tender mercies are over all His works.
Psalm 145:8-9

Date: _____

Name: _____

Home Phone: _____

Cell Phone: _____

Email: _____

Personal Prayer Concerns

_____
_____
_____
_____
_____
_____
_____

This form is for prayer requests that are personal to you and your journey in First Place for Health. Please complete and have it ready to turn in when you arrive at your group meeting.

PRAYER PARTNER   WEEK 6

The Lord is good, a refuge in times of trouble. He cares for those who trust in him. Nahum 1:7

Date: _____

Name: _____

Home Phone: _____

Cell Phone: _____

Email: _____

Personal Prayer Concerns

_____

_____

_____

_____

_____

_____

_____

This form is for prayer requests that are personal to you and your journey in First Place for Health. Please complete and have it ready to turn in when you arrive at your group meeting.

PRAYER PARTNER   WEEK 7

For you know the grace of our Lord Jesus Christ, that though he was rich, yet f or your sake he became poor, so that you through his poverty might become rich.
2 Corinthians 8:9

Date: _____

Name: _____

Home Phone: _____

Cell Phone: _____

Email: _____

Personal Prayer Concerns

_____

_____

_____

_____

_____

_____

_____

_____

This form is for prayer requests that are personal to you and your journey in First Place for Health. Please complete and have it ready to turn in when you arrive at your group meeting.

PRAYER PARTNER   WEEK 8

For you shall go out in joy and be led forth in peace; the mountains and the hills before you shall break forth into singing, and all the trees of the field shall clap their hands.
Isaiah 55:12

Date: _____

Name: _____

Home Phone: _____

Cell Phone: _____

Email: _____

Personal Prayer Concern

_____

_____

_____

_____

_____

_____

_____

This form is for prayer requests that are personal to you and your journey in First Place for Health. Please complete and have it ready to turn in when you arrive at your group meeting.

PRAYER PARTNER WEEK 9

Date:

Name:

Home Phone:

Cell Phone:

Email:

Personal Prayer Concerns

_____

_____

_____

_____

_____

_____

_____

This form is for prayer requests that are personal to you and your journey in First Place for Health. Please complete and have it ready to turn in when you arrive at your group meeting.

LIVE IT TRACKER

Name: _____

My activity goal for next week:
○ None   ○ <30 min/day   ○ 30-60 min/day

My food goal for next week: _____

Date: _____ Week #: _____

loss/gain _____ Calorie Range: _____

My week at a glance:
○ Great   ○ So-so   ○ Not so great

Activity level:
○ None   ○ <30 min/day   ○ 30-60 min/day

RECOMMENDED DAILY AMOUNT OF FOOD FROM EACH GROUP

GROUP	DAILY CALORIES							
	1300-1400	1500-1600	1700-1800	1900-2000	2100-2200	2300-2400	2500-2600	2700-2800
Fruits	1.5 – 2 c.	1.5 – 2 c.	1.5 – 2 c.	2 – 2.5 c.	2 – 2.5 c.	2.5 – 3.5 c.	3.5 – 4.5 c.	3.5 – 4.5 c.
Vegetables	1.5 – 2 c.	2 – 2.5 c.	2.5 – 3 c.	2.5 – 3 c.	3 – 3.5 c.	3.5 – 4.5 c.	4.5 – 5 c.	4.5 – 5 c.
Grains	5 oz eq.	5-6 oz eq.	6-7 oz eq.	6-7 oz eq.	7-8 oz eq.	8-9 oz eq.	9-10 oz eq.	10-11 oz eq.
Dairy	2-3 c.	3 c.	3 c.	3 c.	3 c.	3 c.	3 c.	3 c.
Protein	4 oz eq.	5 oz eq.	5-5.5 oz eq.	5.5-6.5 oz eq.	6.5-7 oz eq.	7-7.5 oz eq.	7-7.5 oz eq.	7.5-8 oz eq.
Healthy Oils & Other Fats	4 tsp.	5 tsp.	5 tsp.	6 tsp.	6 tsp.	7 tsp.	8 tsp.	8 tsp.
Water & Super Beverages*	Women: 9 c. Men: 13 c.	Women: 9 c. Men: 13 c.	Women: 9 c. Men: 13 c.	Women: 9 c. Men: 13 c.	Women: 9 c. Men: 13 c.	Women: 9 c. Men: 13 c.	Women: 9 c. Men: 13 c.	Women: 9 c. Men: 13 c.

*May count up to 3 cups caffeinated tea or coffee toward goal

DAILY FOOD GROUP TRACKER

GROUP	FRUITS	VEGETABLES	GRAINS	PROTEIN	DAIRY	HEALTHY OILS & OTHER FATS	WATER & SUPER BEVERAGES
① Estimate Total							
② Estimate Total							
③ Estimate Total							
④ Estimate Total							
⑤ Estimate Total							
⑥ Estimate Total							
⑦ Estimate Total							

FOOD CHOICES   DAY ❶

Breakfast: _____
Lunch: _____
Dinner: _____
Snacks: _____

PHYSICAL ACTIVITY   steps/miles/minutes: _____

description: _____

SPIRITUAL ACTIVITY

description: _____

FOOD CHOICES — DAY 2
Breakfast: _____
Lunch: _____
Dinner: _____
Snacks: _____

PHYSICAL ACTIVITY steps/miles/minutes: _____
description: _____

SPIRITUAL ACTIVITY
description: _____

FOOD CHOICES — DAY 3
Breakfast: _____
Lunch: _____
Dinner: _____
Snacks: _____

PHYSICAL ACTIVITY steps/miles/minutes: _____
description: _____

SPIRITUAL ACTIVITY
description: _____

FOOD CHOICES — DAY 4
Breakfast: _____
Lunch: _____
Dinner: _____
Snacks: _____

PHYSICAL ACTIVITY steps/miles/minutes: _____
description: _____

SPIRITUAL ACTIVITY
description: _____

FOOD CHOICES — DAY 5
Breakfast: _____
Lunch: _____
Dinner: _____
Snacks: _____

PHYSICAL ACTIVITY steps/miles/minutes: _____
description: _____

SPIRITUAL ACTIVITY
description: _____

FOOD CHOICES — DAY 6
Breakfast: _____
Lunch: _____
Dinner: _____
Snacks: _____

PHYSICAL ACTIVITY steps/miles/minutes: _____
description: _____

SPIRITUAL ACTIVITY
description: _____

FOOD CHOICES — DAY 7
Breakfast: _____
Lunch: _____
Dinner: _____
Snacks: _____

PHYSICAL ACTIVITY steps/miles/minutes: _____
description: _____

SPIRITUAL ACTIVITY
description: _____

LIVE IT TRACKER

Name: _____ Date: _____ Week #: _____

My activity goal for next week:
○ None ○ <30 min/day ○ 30-60 min/day

loss/gain _____ Calorie Range: _____

My week at a glance:
○ Great ○ So-so ○ Not so great

My food goal for next week: _____

Activity level:
○ None ○ <30 min/day ○ 30-60 min/day

RECOMMENDED DAILY AMOUNT OF FOOD FROM EACH GROUP

GROUP	DAILY CALORIES							
	1300-1400	1500-1600	1700-1800	1900-2000	2100-2200	2300-2400	2500-2600	2700-2800
Fruits	1.5 – 2 c.	1.5 – 2 c.	1.5 – 2 c.	2 – 2.5 c.	2 – 2.5 c.	2.5 – 3.5 c.	3.5 – 4.5 c.	3.5 – 4.5 c.
Vegetables	1.5 – 2 c.	2 – 2.5 c.	2.5 – 3 c.	2.5 – 3 c.	3 – 3.5 c.	3.5 – 4.5 c.	4.5 – 5 c.	4.5 – 5 c.
Grains	5 oz eq.	5-6 oz eq.	6-7 oz eq.	6-7 oz eq.	7-8 oz eq.	8-9 oz eq.	9-10 oz eq.	10-11 oz eq.
Dairy	2-3 c.	3 c.	3 c.	3 c.	3 c.	3 c.	3 c.	3 c.
Protein	4 oz eq.	5 oz eq.	5-5.5 oz eq.	5.5-6.5 oz eq.	6.5-7 oz eq.	7-7.5 oz eq.	7-7.5 oz eq.	7.5-8 oz eq.
Healthy Oils & Other Fats	4 tsp.	5 tsp.	5 tsp.	6 tsp.	6 tsp.	7 tsp.	8 tsp.	8 tsp.
Water & Super Beverages*	Women: 9 c. Men: 13 c.	Women: 9 c. Men: 13 c.	Women: 9 c. Men: 13 c.	Women: 9 c. Men: 13 c.	Women: 9 c. Men: 13 c.	Women: 9 c. Men: 13 c.	Women: 9 c. Men: 13 c.	Women: 9 c. Men: 13 c.

*May count up to 3 cups caffeinated tea or coffee toward goal

DAILY FOOD GROUP TRACKER

	GROUP	FRUITS	VEGETABLES	GRAINS	PROTEIN	DAIRY	HEALTHY OILS & OTHER FATS	WATER & SUPER BEVERAGES
1	Estimate Total							
2	Estimate Total							
3	Estimate Total							
4	Estimate Total							
5	Estimate Total							
6	Estimate Total							
7	Estimate Total							

FOOD CHOICES   DAY 1

Breakfast: _____
Lunch: _____
Dinner: _____
Snacks: _____

PHYSICAL ACTIVITY steps/miles/minutes: _____
description: _____

SPIRITUAL ACTIVITY
description: _____

FOOD CHOICES — DAY 2

Breakfast: _____
Lunch: _____
Dinner: _____
Snacks: _____

PHYSICAL ACTIVITY   steps/miles/minutes: _____
description: _____

SPIRITUAL ACTIVITY
description: _____

FOOD CHOICES — DAY 3

Breakfast: _____
Lunch: _____
Dinner: _____
Snacks: _____

PHYSICAL ACTIVITY   steps/miles/minutes: _____
description: _____

SPIRITUAL ACTIVITY
description: _____

FOOD CHOICES — DAY 4

Breakfast: _____
Lunch: _____
Dinner: _____
Snacks: _____

PHYSICAL ACTIVITY   steps/miles/minutes: _____
description: _____

SPIRITUAL ACTIVITY
description: _____

FOOD CHOICES — DAY 5

Breakfast: _____
Lunch: _____
Dinner: _____
Snacks: _____

PHYSICAL ACTIVITY   steps/miles/minutes: _____
description: _____

SPIRITUAL ACTIVITY
description: _____

FOOD CHOICES — DAY 6

Breakfast: _____
Lunch: _____
Dinner: _____
Snacks: _____

PHYSICAL ACTIVITY   steps/miles/minutes: _____
description: _____

SPIRITUAL ACTIVITY
description: _____

FOOD CHOICES — DAY 7

Breakfast: _____
Lunch: _____
Dinner: _____
Snacks: _____

PHYSICAL ACTIVITY   steps/miles/minutes: _____
description: _____

SPIRITUAL ACTIVITY
description: _____

LIVE IT TRACKER

Name: _____

My activity goal for next week:
○ None ○ <30 min/day ○ 30-60 min/day

My food goal for next week: _____

Date: _____ Week #: _____

loss/gain _____ Calorie Range: _____

My week at a glance:
○ Great ○ So-so ○ Not so great

Activity level:
○ None ○ <30 min/day ○ 30-60 min/day

RECOMMENDED DAILY AMOUNT OF FOOD FROM EACH GROUP

GROUP	DAILY CALORIES							
	1300-1400	1500-1600	1700-1800	1900-2000	2100-2200	2300-2400	2500-2600	2700-2800
Fruits	1.5 – 2 c.	1.5 – 2 c.	1.5 – 2 c.	2 – 2.5 c.	2 – 2.5 c.	2.5 – 3.5 c.	3.5 – 4.5 c.	3.5 – 4.5 c.
Vegetables	1.5 – 2 c.	2 – 2.5 c.	2.5 – 3 c.	2.5 – 3 c.	3 – 3.5 c.	3.5 – 4.5 c.	4.5 – 5 c.	4.5 – 5 c.
Grains	5 oz eq.	5-6 oz eq.	6-7 oz eq.	6-7 oz eq.	7-8 oz eq.	8-9 oz eq.	9-10 oz eq.	10-11 oz eq.
Dairy	2-3 c.	3 c.	3 c.	3 c.	3 c.	3 c.	3 c.	3 c.
Protein	4 oz eq.	5 oz eq.	5-5.5 oz eq.	5.5-6.5 oz eq.	6.5-7 oz eq.	7-7.5 oz eq.	7-7.5 oz eq.	7.5-8 oz eq.
Healthy Oils & Other Fats	4 tsp.	5 tsp.	5 tsp.	6 tsp.	6 tsp.	7 tsp.	8 tsp.	8 tsp.
Water & Super Beverages*	Women: 9 c. Men: 13 c.	Women: 9 c. Men: 13 c.	Women: 9 c. Men: 13 c.	Women: 9 c. Men: 13 c.	Women: 9 c. Men: 13 c.	Women: 9 c. Men: 13 c.	Women: 9 c. Men: 13 c.	Women: 9 c. Men: 13 c.

*May count up to 3 cups caffeinated tea or coffee toward goal

DAILY FOOD GROUP TRACKER

GROUP	FRUITS	VEGETABLES	GRAINS	PROTEIN	DAIRY	HEALTHY OILS & OTHER FATS	WATER & SUPER BEVERAGES
❶ Estimate Total							
❷ Estimate Total							
❸ Estimate Total							
❹ Estimate Total							
❺ Estimate Total							
❻ Estimate Total							
❼ Estimate Total							

FOOD CHOICES   DAY ❶

Breakfast: _____
Lunch: _____
Dinner: _____
Snacks: _____

PHYSICAL ACTIVITY   steps/miles/minutes: _____

description: _____

SPIRITUAL ACTIVITY

description: _____

FOOD CHOICES — DAY 2

Breakfast: _____
Lunch: _____
Dinner: _____
Snacks: _____

PHYSICAL ACTIVITY steps/miles/minutes: _____
description: _____

SPIRITUAL ACTIVITY
description: _____

FOOD CHOICES — DAY 3

Breakfast: _____
Lunch: _____
Dinner: _____
Snacks: _____

PHYSICAL ACTIVITY steps/miles/minutes: _____
description: _____

SPIRITUAL ACTIVITY
description: _____

FOOD CHOICES — DAY 4

Breakfast: _____
Lunch: _____
Dinner: _____
Snacks: _____

PHYSICAL ACTIVITY steps/miles/minutes: _____
description: _____

SPIRITUAL ACTIVITY
description: _____

FOOD CHOICES — DAY 5

Breakfast: _____
Lunch: _____
Dinner: _____
Snacks: _____

PHYSICAL ACTIVITY steps/miles/minutes: _____
description: _____

SPIRITUAL ACTIVITY
description: _____

FOOD CHOICES — DAY 6

Breakfast: _____
Lunch: _____
Dinner: _____
Snacks: _____

PHYSICAL ACTIVITY steps/miles/minutes: _____
description: _____

SPIRITUAL ACTIVITY
description: _____

FOOD CHOICES — DAY 7

Breakfast: _____
Lunch: _____
Dinner: _____
Snacks: _____

PHYSICAL ACTIVITY steps/miles/minutes: _____
description: _____

SPIRITUAL ACTIVITY
description: _____

LIVE IT TRACKER

Name: _____ Date: _____ Week #: _____

My activity goal for next week:
○ None   ○ <30 min/day   ○ 30-60 min/day

loss/gain _____   Calorie Range: _____

My week at a glance:
○ Great   ○ So-so   ○ Not so great

My food goal for next week: _____

Activity level:
○ None   ○ <30 min/day   ○ 30-60 min/day

RECOMMENDED DAILY AMOUNT OF FOOD FROM EACH GROUP

GROUP	DAILY CALORIES							
	1300-1400	1500-1600	1700-1800	1900-2000	2100-2200	2300-2400	2500-2600	2700-2800
Fruits	1.5 – 2 c.	1.5 – 2 c.	1.5 – 2 c.	2 – 2.5 c.	2 – 2.5 c.	2.5 – 3.5 c.	3.5 – 4.5 c.	3.5 – 4.5 c.
Vegetables	1.5 – 2 c.	2 – 2.5 c.	2.5 – 3 c.	2.5 – 3 c.	3 – 3.5 c.	3.5 – 4.5 c.	4.5 – 5 c.	4.5 – 5 c.
Grains	5 oz eq.	5-6 oz eq.	6-7 oz eq.	6-7 oz eq.	7-8 oz eq.	8-9 oz eq.	9-10 oz eq.	10-11 oz eq.
Dairy	2-3 c.	3 c.	3 c.	3 c.	3 c.	3 c.	3 c.	3 c.
Protein	4 oz eq.	5 oz eq.	5-5.5 oz eq.	5.5-6.5 oz eq.	6.5-7 oz eq.	7-7.5 oz eq.	7-7.5 oz eq.	7.5-8 oz eq.
Healthy Oils & Other Fats	4 tsp.	5 tsp.	5 tsp.	6 tsp.	6 tsp.	7 tsp.	8 tsp.	8 tsp.
Water & Super Beverages*	Women: 9 c. Men: 13 c.	Women: 9 c. Men: 13 c.	Women: 9 c. Men: 13 c.	Women: 9 c. Men: 13 c.	Women: 9 c. Men: 13 c.	Women: 9 c. Men: 13 c.	Women: 9 c. Men: 13 c.	Women: 9 c. Men: 13 c.

*May count up to 3 cups caffeinated tea or coffee toward goal

DAILY FOOD GROUP TRACKER

GROUP	FRUITS	VEGETABLES	GRAINS	PROTEIN	DAIRY	HEALTHY OILS & OTHER FATS	WATER & SUPER BEVERAGES
❶ Estimate Total							
❷ Estimate Total							
❸ Estimate Total							
❹ Estimate Total							
❺ Estimate Total							
❻ Estimate Total							
❼ Estimate Total							

FOOD CHOICES   DAY ❶

Breakfast: _____
Lunch: _____
Dinner: _____
Snacks: _____

PHYSICAL ACTIVITY   steps/miles/minutes: _____
description: _____

SPIRITUAL ACTIVITY
description: _____

DAY 2

FOOD CHOICES
Breakfast: _____
Lunch: _____
Dinner: _____
Snacks: _____

PHYSICAL ACTIVITY steps/miles/minutes: _____
description: _____

SPIRITUAL ACTIVITY
description: _____

DAY 3

FOOD CHOICES
Breakfast: _____
Lunch: _____
Dinner: _____
Snacks: _____

PHYSICAL ACTIVITY steps/miles/minutes: _____
description: _____

SPIRITUAL ACTIVITY
description: _____

DAY 4

FOOD CHOICES
Breakfast: _____
Lunch: _____
Dinner: _____
Snacks: _____

PHYSICAL ACTIVITY steps/miles/minutes: _____
description: _____

SPIRITUAL ACTIVITY
description: _____

DAY 5

FOOD CHOICES
Breakfast: _____
Lunch: _____
Dinner: _____
Snacks: _____

PHYSICAL ACTIVITY steps/miles/minutes: _____
description: _____

SPIRITUAL ACTIVITY
description: _____

DAY 6

FOOD CHOICES
Breakfast: _____
Lunch: _____
Dinner: _____
Snacks: _____

PHYSICAL ACTIVITY steps/miles/minutes: _____
description: _____

SPIRITUAL ACTIVITY
description: _____

DAY 7

FOOD CHOICES
Breakfast: _____
Lunch: _____
Dinner: _____
Snacks: _____

PHYSICAL ACTIVITY steps/miles/minutes: _____
description: _____

SPIRITUAL ACTIVITY
description: _____

LIVE IT TRACKER

Name: _____

Date: _____ Week #: _____

My activity goal for next week:
○ None ○ <30 min/day ○ 30-60 min/day

loss/gain _____ Calorie Range: _____

My week at a glance:
○ Great ○ So-so ○ Not so great

My food goal for next week: _____

Activity level:
○ None ○ <30 min/day ○ 30-60 min/day

RECOMMENDED DAILY AMOUNT OF FOOD FROM EACH GROUP

GROUP	DAILY CALORIES							
	1300-1400	1500-1600	1700-1800	1900-2000	2100-2200	2300-2400	2500-2600	2700-2800
Fruits	1.5 – 2 c.	1.5 – 2 c.	1.5 – 2 c.	2 – 2.5 c.	2 – 2.5 c.	2.5 – 3.5 c.	3.5 – 4.5 c.	3.5 – 4.5 c.
Vegetables	1.5 – 2 c.	2 – 2.5 c.	2.5 – 3 c.	2.5 – 3 c.	3 – 3.5 c.	3.5 – 4.5 c.	4.5 – 5 c.	4.5 – 5 c.
Grains	5 oz eq.	5-6 oz eq.	6-7 oz eq.	6-7 oz eq.	7-8 oz eq.	8-9 oz eq.	9-10 oz eq.	10-11 oz eq.
Dairy	2-3 c.	3 c.	3 c.	3 c.	3 c.	3 c.	3 c.	3 c.
Protein	4 oz eq.	5 oz eq.	5-5.5 oz eq.	5.5-6.5 oz eq.	6.5-7 oz eq.	7-7.5 oz eq.	7-7.5 oz eq.	7.5-8 oz eq.
Healthy Oils & Other Fats	4 tsp.	5 tsp.	5 tsp.	6 tsp.	6 tsp.	7 tsp.	8 tsp.	8 tsp.
Water & Super Beverages*	Women: 9 c. Men: 13 c.	Women: 9 c. Men: 13 c.	Women: 9 c. Men: 13 c.	Women: 9 c. Men: 13 c.	Women: 9 c. Men: 13 c.	Women: 9 c. Men: 13 c.	Women: 9 c. Men: 13 c.	Women: 9 c. Men: 13 c.

*May count up to 3 cups caffeinated tea or coffee toward goal

DAILY FOOD GROUP TRACKER

GROUP	FRUITS	VEGETABLES	GRAINS	PROTEIN	DAIRY	HEALTHY OILS & OTHER FATS	WATER & SUPER BEVERAGES
❶ Estimate Total							
❷ Estimate Total							
❸ Estimate Total							
❹ Estimate Total							
❺ Estimate Total							
❻ Estimate Total							
❼ Estimate Total							

FOOD CHOICES   DAY ❶

Breakfast: _____
Lunch: _____
Dinner: _____
Snacks: _____

PHYSICAL ACTIVITY   steps/miles/minutes: _____
description: _____

SPIRITUAL ACTIVITY
description: _____

FOOD CHOICES — DAY 2

Breakfast: _____
Lunch: _____
Dinner: _____
Snacks: _____

PHYSICAL ACTIVITY steps/miles/minutes: _____
description: _____

SPIRITUAL ACTIVITY
description: _____

FOOD CHOICES — DAY 3

Breakfast: _____
Lunch: _____
Dinner: _____
Snacks: _____

PHYSICAL ACTIVITY steps/miles/minutes: _____
description: _____

SPIRITUAL ACTIVITY
description: _____

FOOD CHOICES — DAY 4

Breakfast: _____
Lunch: _____
Dinner: _____
Snacks: _____

PHYSICAL ACTIVITY steps/miles/minutes: _____
description: _____

SPIRITUAL ACTIVITY
description: _____

FOOD CHOICES — DAY 5

Breakfast: _____
Lunch: _____
Dinner: _____
Snacks: _____

PHYSICAL ACTIVITY steps/miles/minutes: _____
description: _____

SPIRITUAL ACTIVITY
description: _____

FOOD CHOICES — DAY 6

Breakfast: _____
Lunch: _____
Dinner: _____
Snacks: _____

PHYSICAL ACTIVITY steps/miles/minutes: _____
description: _____

SPIRITUAL ACTIVITY
description: _____

FOOD CHOICES — DAY 7

Breakfast: _____
Lunch: _____
Dinner: _____
Snacks: _____

PHYSICAL ACTIVITY steps/miles/minutes: _____
description: _____

SPIRITUAL ACTIVITY
description: _____

LIVE IT TRACKER

Name: _____

Date: _____ Week #: _____

My activity goal for next week:
○ None ○ <30 min/day ○ 30-60 min/day

loss/gain _____ Calorie Range: _____

My week at a glance:
○ Great ○ So-so ○ Not so great

My food goal for next week: _____

Activity level:
○ None ○ <30 min/day ○ 30-60 min/day

RECOMMENDED DAILY AMOUNT OF FOOD FROM EACH GROUP

GROUP	DAILY CALORIES							
	1300-1400	1500-1600	1700-1800	1900-2000	2100-2200	2300-2400	2500-2600	2700-2800
Fruits	1.5 – 2 c.	1.5 – 2 c.	1.5 – 2 c.	2 – 2.5 c.	2 – 2.5 c.	2.5 – 3.5 c.	3.5 – 4.5 c.	3.5 – 4.5 c.
Vegetables	1.5 – 2 c.	2 – 2.5 c.	2.5 – 3 c.	2.5 – 3 c.	3 – 3.5 c.	3.5 – 4.5 c.	4.5 – 5 c.	4.5 – 5 c.
Grains	5 oz eq.	5-6 oz eq.	6-7 oz eq.	6-7 oz eq.	7-8 oz eq.	8-9 oz eq.	9-10 oz eq.	10-11 oz eq.
Dairy	2-3 c.	3 c.	3 c.	3 c.	3 c.	3 c.	3 c.	3 c.
Protein	4 oz eq.	5 oz eq.	5-5.5 oz eq.	5.5-6.5 oz eq.	6.5-7 oz eq.	7-7.5 oz eq.	7-7.5 oz eq.	7.5-8 oz eq.
Healthy Oils & Other Fats	4 tsp.	5 tsp.	5 tsp.	6 tsp.	6 tsp.	7 tsp.	8 tsp.	8 tsp.
Water & Super Beverages*	Women: 9 c. Men: 13 c.	Women: 9 c. Men: 13 c.	Women: 9 c. Men: 13 c.	Women: 9 c. Men: 13 c.	Women: 9 c. Men: 13 c.	Women: 9 c. Men: 13 c.	Women: 9 c. Men: 13 c.	Women: 9 c. Men: 13 c.

*May count up to 3 cups caffeinated tea or coffee toward goal

DAILY FOOD GROUP TRACKER

GROUP	FRUITS	VEGETABLES	GRAINS	PROTEIN	DAIRY	HEALTHY OILS & OTHER FATS	WATER & SUPER BEVERAGES
1 Estimate Total							
2 Estimate Total							
3 Estimate Total							
4 Estimate Total							
5 Estimate Total							
6 Estimate Total							
7 Estimate Total							

FOOD CHOICES — DAY 1

Breakfast: _____
Lunch: _____
Dinner: _____
Snacks: _____

PHYSICAL ACTIVITY   steps/miles/minutes: _____
description: _____

SPIRITUAL ACTIVITY
description: _____

DAY ❷

FOOD CHOICES
Breakfast: _____
Lunch: _____
Dinner: _____
Snacks: _____

PHYSICAL ACTIVITY steps/miles/minutes: _____
description: _____

SPIRITUAL ACTIVITY
description: _____

DAY ❸

FOOD CHOICES
Breakfast: _____
Lunch: _____
Dinner: _____
Snacks: _____

PHYSICAL ACTIVITY steps/miles/minutes: _____
description: _____

SPIRITUAL ACTIVITY
description: _____

DAY ❹

FOOD CHOICES
Breakfast: _____
Lunch: _____
Dinner: _____
Snacks: _____

PHYSICAL ACTIVITY steps/miles/minutes: _____
description: _____

SPIRITUAL ACTIVITY
description: _____

DAY ❺

FOOD CHOICES
Breakfast: _____
Lunch: _____
Dinner: _____
Snacks: _____

PHYSICAL ACTIVITY steps/miles/minutes: _____
description: _____

SPIRITUAL ACTIVITY
description: _____

DAY ❻

FOOD CHOICES
Breakfast: _____
Lunch: _____
Dinner: _____
Snacks: _____

PHYSICAL ACTIVITY steps/miles/minutes: _____
description: _____

SPIRITUAL ACTIVITY
description: _____

DAY ❼

FOOD CHOICES
Breakfast: _____
Lunch: _____
Dinner: _____
Snacks: _____

PHYSICAL ACTIVITY steps/miles/minutes: _____
description: _____

SPIRITUAL ACTIVITY
description: _____

LIVE IT TRACKER

Name: _____

Date: _____ Week #: _____

My activity goal for next week:
○ None ○ <30 min/day ○ 30-60 min/day

loss/gain _____ Calorie Range: _____

My week at a glance:
○ Great ○ So-so ○ Not so great

My food goal for next week: _____

Activity level:
○ None ○ <30 min/day ○ 30-60 min/day

RECOMMENDED DAILY AMOUNT OF FOOD FROM EACH GROUP

GROUP	DAILY CALORIES							
	1300-1400	1500-1600	1700-1800	1900-2000	2100-2200	2300-2400	2500-2600	2700-2800
Fruits	1.5 – 2 c.	1.5 – 2 c.	1.5 – 2 c.	2 – 2.5 c.	2 – 2.5 c.	2.5 – 3.5 c.	3.5 – 4.5 c.	3.5 – 4.5 c.
Vegetables	1.5 – 2 c.	2 – 2.5 c.	2.5 – 3 c.	2.5 – 3 c.	3 – 3.5 c.	3.5 – 4.5 c.	4.5 – 5 c.	4.5 – 5 c.
Grains	5 oz eq.	5-6 oz eq.	6-7 oz eq.	6-7 oz eq.	7-8 oz eq.	8-9 oz eq.	9-10 oz eq.	10-11 oz eq.
Dairy	2-3 c.	3 c.	3 c.	3 c.	3 c.	3 c.	3 c.	3 c.
Protein	4 oz eq.	5 oz eq.	5-5.5 oz eq.	5.5-6.5 oz eq.	6.5-7 oz eq.	7-7.5 oz eq.	7-7.5 oz eq.	7.5-8 oz eq.
Healthy Oils & Other Fats	4 tsp.	5 tsp.	5 tsp.	6 tsp.	6 tsp.	7 tsp.	8 tsp.	8 tsp.
Water & Super Beverages*	Women: 9 c. Men: 13 c.	Women: 9 c. Men: 13 c.	Women: 9 c. Men: 13 c.	Women: 9 c. Men: 13 c.	Women: 9 c. Men: 13 c.	Women: 9 c. Men: 13 c.	Women: 9 c. Men: 13 c.	Women: 9 c. Men: 13 c.

*May count up to 3 cups caffeinated tea or coffee toward goal

DAILY FOOD GROUP TRACKER

GROUP	FRUITS	VEGETABLES	GRAINS	PROTEIN	DAIRY	HEALTHY OILS & OTHER FATS	WATER & SUPER BEVERAGES
① Estimate Total							
② Estimate Total							
③ Estimate Total							
④ Estimate Total							
⑤ Estimate Total							
⑥ Estimate Total							
⑦ Estimate Total							

FOOD CHOICES   DAY ❶

Breakfast: _____
Lunch: _____
Dinner: _____
Snacks: _____

PHYSICAL ACTIVITY   steps/miles/minutes: _____
description: _____

SPIRITUAL ACTIVITY
description: _____

FOOD CHOICES — DAY 2
Breakfast: _____
Lunch: _____
Dinner: _____
Snacks: _____

PHYSICAL ACTIVITY steps/miles/minutes: _____
description: _____

SPIRITUAL ACTIVITY
description: _____

FOOD CHOICES — DAY 3
Breakfast: _____
Lunch: _____
Dinner: _____
Snacks: _____

PHYSICAL ACTIVITY steps/miles/minutes: _____
description: _____

SPIRITUAL ACTIVITY
description: _____

FOOD CHOICES — DAY 4
Breakfast: _____
Lunch: _____
Dinner: _____
Snacks: _____

PHYSICAL ACTIVITY steps/miles/minutes: _____
description: _____

SPIRITUAL ACTIVITY
description: _____

FOOD CHOICES — DAY 5
Breakfast: _____
Lunch: _____
Dinner: _____
Snacks: _____

PHYSICAL ACTIVITY steps/miles/minutes: _____
description: _____

SPIRITUAL ACTIVITY
description: _____

FOOD CHOICES — DAY 6
Breakfast: _____
Lunch: _____
Dinner: _____
Snacks: _____

PHYSICAL ACTIVITY steps/miles/minutes: _____
description: _____

SPIRITUAL ACTIVITY
description: _____

FOOD CHOICES — DAY 7
Breakfast: _____
Lunch: _____
Dinner: _____
Snacks: _____

PHYSICAL ACTIVITY steps/miles/minutes: _____
description: _____

SPIRITUAL ACTIVITY
description: _____

LIVE IT TRACKER

Name: _____

Date: _____ Week #: _____

My activity goal for next week:
○ None ○ <30 min/day ○ 30-60 min/day

loss/gain _____ Calorie Range: _____

My food goal for next week: _____

My week at a glance:
○ Great ○ So-so ○ Not so great

Activity level:
○ None ○ <30 min/day ○ 30-60 min/day

RECOMMENDED DAILY AMOUNT OF FOOD FROM EACH GROUP

GROUP	DAILY CALORIES							
	1300-1400	1500-1600	1700-1800	1900-2000	2100-2200	2300-2400	2500-2600	2700-2800
Fruits	1.5 – 2 c.	1.5 – 2 c.	1.5 – 2 c.	2 – 2.5 c.	2 – 2.5 c.	2.5 – 3.5 c.	3.5 – 4.5 c.	3.5 – 4.5 c.
Vegetables	1.5 – 2 c.	2 – 2.5 c.	2.5 – 3 c.	2.5 – 3 c.	3 – 3.5 c.	3.5 – 4.5 c.	4.5 – 5 c.	4.5 – 5 c.
Grains	5 oz eq.	5-6 oz eq.	6-7 oz eq.	6-7 oz eq.	7-8 oz eq.	8-9 oz eq.	9-10 oz eq.	10-11 oz eq.
Dairy	2-3 c.	3 c.	3 c.	3 c.	3 c.	3 c.	3 c.	3 c.
Protein	4 oz eq.	5 oz eq.	5-5.5 oz eq.	5.5-6.5 oz eq.	6.5-7 oz eq.	7-7.5 oz eq.	7-7.5 oz eq.	7.5-8 oz eq.
Healthy Oils & Other Fats	4 tsp.	5 tsp.	5 tsp.	6 tsp.	6 tsp.	7 tsp.	8 tsp.	8 tsp.
Water & Super Beverages*	Women: 9 c. Men: 13 c.	Women: 9 c. Men: 13 c.	Women: 9 c. Men: 13 c.	Women: 9 c. Men: 13 c.	Women: 9 c. Men: 13 c.	Women: 9 c. Men: 13 c.	Women: 9 c. Men: 13 c.	Women: 9 c. Men: 13 c.

*May count up to 3 cups caffeinated tea or coffee toward goal

DAILY FOOD GROUP TRACKER

	GROUP	FRUITS	VEGETABLES	GRAINS	PROTEIN	DAIRY	HEALTHY OILS & OTHER FATS	WATER & SUPER BEVERAGES
1	Estimate Total							
2	Estimate Total							
3	Estimate Total							
4	Estimate Total							
5	Estimate Total							
6	Estimate Total							
7	Estimate Total							

FOOD CHOICES   DAY 1

Breakfast: _____
Lunch: _____
Dinner: _____
Snacks: _____

PHYSICAL ACTIVITY   steps/miles/minutes: _____
description: _____

SPIRITUAL ACTIVITY
description: _____

DAY 2

FOOD CHOICES
Breakfast: _____
Lunch: _____
Dinner: _____
Snacks: _____

PHYSICAL ACTIVITY steps/miles/minutes: _____
description: _____

SPIRITUAL ACTIVITY
description: _____

DAY 3

FOOD CHOICES
Breakfast: _____
Lunch: _____
Dinner: _____
Snacks: _____

PHYSICAL ACTIVITY steps/miles/minutes: _____
description: _____

SPIRITUAL ACTIVITY
description: _____

DAY 4

FOOD CHOICES
Breakfast: _____
Lunch: _____
Dinner: _____
Snacks: _____

PHYSICAL ACTIVITY steps/miles/minutes: _____
description: _____

SPIRITUAL ACTIVITY
description: _____

DAY 5

FOOD CHOICES
Breakfast: _____
Lunch: _____
Dinner: _____
Snacks: _____

PHYSICAL ACTIVITY steps/miles/minutes: _____
description: _____

SPIRITUAL ACTIVITY
description: _____

DAY 6

FOOD CHOICES
Breakfast: _____
Lunch: _____
Dinner: _____
Snacks: _____

PHYSICAL ACTIVITY steps/miles/minutes: _____
description: _____

SPIRITUAL ACTIVITY
description: _____

DAY 7

FOOD CHOICES
Breakfast: _____
Lunch: _____
Dinner: _____
Snacks: _____

PHYSICAL ACTIVITY steps/miles/minutes: _____
description: _____

SPIRITUAL ACTIVITY
description: _____

LIVE IT TRACKER

Name: _____

Date: _____ Week #: _____

My activity goal for next week:
○ None ○ <30 min/day ○ 30-60 min/day

loss/gain _____ Calorie Range: _____

My week at a glance:
○ Great ○ So-so ○ Not so great

My food goal for next week: _____

Activity level:
○ None ○ <30 min/day ○ 30-60 min/day

RECOMMENDED DAILY AMOUNT OF FOOD FROM EACH GROUP

GROUP	DAILY CALORIES							
	1300-1400	1500-1600	1700-1800	1900-2000	2100-2200	2300-2400	2500-2600	2700-2800
Fruits	1.5 – 2 c.	1.5 – 2 c.	1.5 – 2 c.	2 – 2.5 c.	2 – 2.5 c.	2.5 – 3.5 c.	3.5 – 4.5 c.	3.5 – 4.5 c.
Vegetables	1.5 – 2 c.	2 – 2.5 c.	2.5 – 3 c.	2.5 – 3 c.	3 – 3.5 c.	3.5 – 4.5 c.	4.5 – 5 c.	4.5 – 5 c.
Grains	5 oz eq.	5-6 oz eq.	6-7 oz eq.	6-7 oz eq.	7-8 oz eq.	8-9 oz eq.	9-10 oz eq.	10-11 oz eq.
Dairy	2-3 c.	3 c.	3 c.	3 c.	3 c.	3 c.	3 c.	3 c.
Protein	4 oz eq.	5 oz eq.	5-5.5 oz eq.	5.5-6.5 oz eq.	6.5-7 oz eq.	7-7.5 oz eq.	7-7.5 oz eq.	7.5-8 oz eq.
Healthy Oils & Other Fats	4 tsp.	5 tsp.	5 tsp.	6 tsp.	6 tsp.	7 tsp.	8 tsp.	8 tsp.
Water & Super Beverages*	Women: 9 c. Men: 13 c.	Women: 9 c. Men: 13 c.	Women: 9 c. Men: 13 c.	Women: 9 c. Men: 13 c.	Women: 9 c. Men: 13 c.	Women: 9 c. Men: 13 c.	Women: 9 c. Men: 13 c.	Women: 9 c. Men: 13 c.

*May count up to 3 cups caffeinated tea or coffee toward goal

DAILY FOOD GROUP TRACKER

GROUP	FRUITS	VEGETABLES	GRAINS	PROTEIN	DAIRY	HEALTHY OILS & OTHER FATS	WATER & SUPER BEVERAGES
① Estimate Total							
② Estimate Total							
③ Estimate Total							
④ Estimate Total							
⑤ Estimate Total							
⑥ Estimate Total							
⑦ Estimate Total							

FOOD CHOICES — DAY ❶

Breakfast: _____
Lunch: _____
Dinner: _____
Snacks: _____

PHYSICAL ACTIVITY   steps/miles/minutes: _____
description: _____

SPIRITUAL ACTIVITY
description: _____

FOOD CHOICES — DAY 2
Breakfast: _____
Lunch: _____
Dinner: _____
Snacks: _____

PHYSICAL ACTIVITY steps/miles/minutes: _____ | **SPIRITUAL ACTIVITY**
description: _____ | description: _____

FOOD CHOICES — DAY 3
Breakfast: _____
Lunch: _____
Dinner: _____
Snacks: _____

PHYSICAL ACTIVITY steps/miles/minutes: _____ | **SPIRITUAL ACTIVITY**
description: _____ | description: _____

FOOD CHOICES — DAY 4
Breakfast: _____
Lunch: _____
Dinner: _____
Snacks: _____

PHYSICAL ACTIVITY steps/miles/minutes: _____ | **SPIRITUAL ACTIVITY**
description: _____ | description: _____

FOOD CHOICES — DAY 5
Breakfast: _____
Lunch: _____
Dinner: _____
Snacks: _____

PHYSICAL ACTIVITY steps/miles/minutes: _____ | **SPIRITUAL ACTIVITY**
description: _____ | description: _____

FOOD CHOICES — DAY 6
Breakfast: _____
Lunch: _____
Dinner: _____
Snacks: _____

PHYSICAL ACTIVITY steps/miles/minutes: _____ | **SPIRITUAL ACTIVITY**
description: _____ | description: _____

FOOD CHOICES — DAY 7
Breakfast: _____
Lunch: _____
Dinner: _____
Snacks: _____

PHYSICAL ACTIVITY steps/miles/minutes: _____ | **SPIRITUAL ACTIVITY**
description: _____ | description: _____

100-MILE CLUB

WALKING			
slowly, 2 mph	30 min =	156 cal =	1 mile
moderately, 3 mph	20 min =	156 cal =	1 mile
very briskly, 4 mph	15 min =	156 cal =	1 mile
speed walking	10 min =	156 cal =	1 mile
up stairs	13 min =	159 cal =	1 mile
RUNNING / JOGGING			
...	10 min =	156 cal =	1 mile
CYCLE OUTDOORS			
slowly, < 10 mph	20 min =	156 cal =	1 mile
light effort, 10-12 mph	12 min =	156 cal =	1 mile
moderate effort, 12-14 mph	10 min =	156 cal =	1 mile
vigorous effort, 14-16 mph	7.5 min =	156 cal =	1 mile
very fast, 16-19 mph	6.5 min =	152 cal =	1 mile
SPORTS ACTIVITIES			
playing tennis (singles)	10 min =	156 cal =	1 mile
swimming			
light to moderate effort	11 min =	152 cal =	1 mile
fast, vigorous effort	7.5 min =	156 cal =	1 mile
softball	15 min =	156 cal =	1 mile
golf	20 min =	156 cal =	1 mile
rollerblading	6.5 min =	152 cal =	1 mile
ice skating	11 min =	152 cal =	1 mile
jumping rope	7.5 min =	156 cal =	1 mile
basketball	12 min =	156 cal =	1 mile
soccer (casual)	15 min =	159 min =	1 mile
AROUND THE HOUSE			
mowing grass	22 min =	156 cal =	1 mile
mopping, sweeping, vacuuming	19.5 min =	155 cal =	1 mile
cooking	40 min =	160 cal =	1 mile
gardening	19 min =	156 cal =	1 mile
housework (general)	35 min =	156 cal =	1 mile

AROUND THE HOUSE			
ironing	45 min =	153 cal =	1 mile
raking leaves	25 min =	150 cal =	1 mile
washing car	23 min =	156 cal =	1 mile
washing dishes	45 min =	153 cal =	1 mile
AT THE GYM			
stair machine	8.5 min =	155 cal =	1 mile
stationary bike			
slowly, 10 mph	30 min =	156 cal =	1 mile
moderately, 10-13 mph	15 min =	156 cal =	1 mile
vigorously, 13-16 mph	7.5 min =	156 cal =	1 mile
briskly, 16-19 mph	6.5 min =	156 cal =	1 mile
elliptical trainer	12 min =	156 cal =	1 mile
weight machines (vigorously)	13 min =	152 cal =	1 mile
aerobics			
low impact	15 min =	156 cal =	1 mile
high impact	12 min =	156 cal =	1 mile
water	20 min =	156 cal =	1 mile
pilates	15 min =	156 cal =	1 mile
raquetball (casual)	15 min =	156 cal =	1 mile
stretching exercises	25 min =	150 cal =	1 mile
weight lifting (also works for weight machines used moderately or gently)	30 min =	156 cal =	1 mile
FAMILY LEISURE			
playing piano	37 min =	155 cal =	1 mile
jumping rope	10 min =	152 cal =	1 mile
skating (moderate)	20 min =	152 cal =	1 mile
swimming			
moderate	17 min =	156 cal =	1 mile
vigorous	10 min =	148 cal =	1 mile
table tennis	25 min =	150 cal =	1 mile
walk / run / play with kids	25 min =	150 cal =	1 mile

Let's Count Our Miles!

Color each circle to represent a mile you've completed.
Watch your progress to that 100 mile marker!

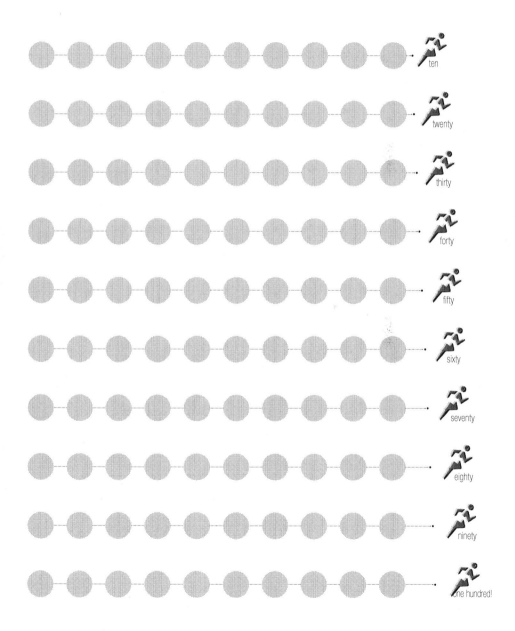

Made in the USA
Middletown, DE
26 March 2022

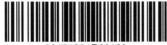